Technical Brief

Number 15

Transition Care for Children With Special Health Needs

Prepared for:
Agency for Healthcare Research and Quality
U.S. Department of Health and Human Services
540 Gaither Road
Rockville, MD 20850
www.ahrq.gov

Contract No. 290-2012-00009-I

Prepared by:
Vanderbilt University Evidence-based Practice Center
Nashville, TN

Investigators:
Melissa McPheeters, Ph.D., M.P.H.
Alaina M. Davis, M.D.
Julie Lounds Taylor, Ph.D., M.A.
Rebekah Flowers Brown, M.D.
Shannon A. Potter, M.L.I.S.
Richard A. Epstein, Jr., Ph.D., M.P.H.

AHRQ Publication No. 14-EHC027-EF
June 2014

This report is based on research conducted by the Vanderbilt University Evidence-based Practice Center (EPC) under contract to the Agency for Healthcare Research and Quality (AHRQ), Rockville, MD (Contract No. 290-2012-00009-I).

The findings and conclusions in this document are those of the author(s), who are responsible for its contents; the findings and conclusions do not necessarily represent the views of AHRQ. Therefore, no statement in this report should be construed as an official position of AHRQ or of the U.S. Department of Health and Human Services.

The information in this report is intended to help health care decisionmakers—patients and providers, health system leaders, and policymakers, among others—make well-informed decisions and thereby improve the quality of health care services. This report is not intended to be a substitute for the application of clinical judgment. Anyone who makes decisions concerning the provision of clinical care should consider this report in the same way as any medical reference and in conjunction with all other pertinent information, i.e., in the context of available resources and circumstances presented by individual patients.

This report may be used, in whole or in part, as the basis for development of clinical practice guidelines and other quality enhancement tools, or as a basis for reimbursement and coverage policies. AHRQ or U.S. Department of Health and Human Services endorsement of such derivative products may not be stated or implied.

This document is in the public domain and may be used and reprinted without permission except those copyrighted materials noted, for which further reproduction is prohibited without the specific permission of copyright holders.

Persons using assistive technology may not be able to fully access information in this report. For assistance contact EffectiveHealthCare@ahrq.hhs.gov.

None of the investigators have any affiliation or financial involvement that conflicts with the material presented in this report.

Suggested citation: McPheeters M, Davis AM, Taylor JL, Brown RF, Potter SA, Epstein RA. Transition Care for Children With Special Health Needs. Technical Brief No. 15 (Prepared by the Vanderbilt University Evidence-based Practice Center under Contract No. 290-2012-00009-I). AHRQ Publication No.14-EHC027-EF. Rockville, MD: Agency for Healthcare Research and Quality. June 2014. www.effectivehealthcare.ahrq.gov/reports/final.cfm.

Preface

The Agency for Healthcare Research and Quality (AHRQ), through its Evidence-based Practice Centers (EPCs), sponsors the development of evidence reports and technology assessments to assist public- and private-sector organizations in their efforts to improve the quality of health care in the United States. The reports and assessments provide organizations with comprehensive, science-based information on common, costly medical conditions and new health care technologies and strategies. The EPCs systematically review the relevant scientific literature on topics assigned to them by AHRQ and conduct additional analyses when appropriate prior to developing their reports and assessments.

This EPC evidence report is a Technical Brief. A Technical Brief is a rapid report, typically on an emerging medical technology, strategy, or intervention. It provides an overview of key issues related to the intervention—for example, current indications, relevant patient populations and subgroups of interest, outcomes measured, and contextual factors that may affect decisions regarding the intervention. Although Technical Briefs generally focus on interventions for which there are limited published data and too few completed protocol-driven studies to support definitive conclusions, the decision to request a Technical Brief is not solely based on the availability of clinical studies. The goals of the Technical Brief are to provide an early objective description of the state of the science, a potential framework for assessing the applications and implications of the intervention, a summary of ongoing research, and information on future research needs. In particular, through the Technical Brief, AHRQ hopes to gain insight on the appropriate conceptual framework and critical issues that will inform future research.

AHRQ expects that the EPC evidence reports and technology assessments will inform individual health plans, providers, and purchasers as well as the health care system as a whole by providing important information to help improve health care quality.

We welcome comments on this Technical Brief. They may be sent by mail to the Task Order Officer named below at: Agency for Healthcare Research and Quality, 540 Gaither Road, Rockville, MD 20850, or by email to epc@ahrq.hhs.gov.

Richard G. Kronick, Ph.D.
Director, Agency for Healthcare Research and Quality

Stephanie Chang, M.D., M.P.H.
Director, EPC Program
Center for Outcomes and Evidence
Agency for Healthcare Research and Quality

Yen-pin Chiang, Ph.D.
Acting Director, Center for Outcomes and Evidence
Agency for Healthcare Research and Quality

Christine Chang, M.D., M.P.H.
Task Order Officer
Center for Outcomes and Evidence
Agency for Healthcare Research and Quality

Acknowledgments

The authors gratefully acknowledge the following individuals for their contributions to this project: Ms. Rebecca Jerome, Ms. Natalie A. Henninger, Ms. Tanya Surawicz, Ms. Sanura Latham, and Ms. Jessica Kimber.

Key Informants

In designing the study questions, the EPC consulted a panel of Key Informants who represent subject experts and end-users of research. Key Informant input can inform key issues related to the topic of the technical brief. Key Informants are not involved in the analysis of the evidence or the writing of the report. Therefore, in the end, study questions, design, methodological approaches and/or conclusions do not necessarily represent the views of individual Key Informants.

Key Informants must disclose any financial conflicts of interest greater than $10,000 and any other relevant business or professional conflicts of interest. Because of their role as end-users, individuals with potential conflicts may be retained. The Task Order Officer and the Evidence-based Practice Center work to balance, manage, or mitigate any conflicts of interest.

The list of Key Informants who participated in developing this report follows:

Michael S. Barr, M.D., M.B.A., FACP
Division of Medical Practice
American College of Physicians
Washington, D.C.

Charles J. Homer, M.D., M.P.H.
Chief Executive Officer and President
National Initiative for Children's Healthcare Quality
Boston, MA

Marie Mann, M.D., M.P.H.
Maternal and Child Health Bureau
Rockville, MD

Elise McMillan, J.D.
Vanderbilt Kennedy Center for Excellence in Developmental Disabilities
Nashville, TN

Cynthia Peacock, M.D., FAAP, FACP
Baylor Transition Medicine Clinic
Houston, TX

Peer Reviewers

Prior to publication of the final evidence report, EPCs sought input from independent Peer reviewers without financial conflicts of interest. However, the conclusions and synthesis of the scientific literature presented in this report does not necessarily represent the views of individual reviewers.

Peer Reviewers must disclose any financial conflicts of interest greater than $10,000 and any other relevant business or professional conflicts of interest. Because of their unique clinical or content expertise, individuals with potential nonfinancial conflicts may be retained. The TOO and the EPC work to balance, manage, or mitigate any potential nonfinancial conflicts of interest identified.

The list of Peer Reviewers follows:

Rachel Annunziato, Ph.D.
Fordham University
Bronx, NY

Michael S. Barr, M.D., M.B.A., FACP
Division of Medical Practice
American College of Physicians
Washington, D.C.

Cecily L. Betz, Ph.D., R.N., FAAN
USC UCEDD at Children's Hospital
Los Angeles, CA

William Carl Cooley, M.D.
Crotched Mountain Rehabilitation Center
Greenfield, NH

Charles J. Homer, M.D., M.P.H.
Chief Executive Officer and President,
National Initiative for Children's Healthcare
Quality
Boston, MA

Marie Mann, M.D., M.P.H.
Maternal and Child Health Bureau
Rockville, MD

Elise McMillan, J.D.
Vanderbilt Kennedy Center for Excellence
in Developmental Disabilities
Nashville, TN

Megumi J. Okumura M.D., M.A.S.
Division of General Pediatrics
Division of General Internal Medicine
University of California San Francisco
San Francisco, CA

Melissa Parisi, Ph.D., M.D.
Intellectual and Developmental Disabilities
Branch
Eunice Kennedy Shriver National Institute
of Child Health and Human Development
National Institutes of Health
Bethesda, MD

Cynthia Peacock, M.D., FAAP, FACP
Baylor Transition Medicine Clinic
Houston, TX

John Reiss, Ph.D., M.A.
Institute for Child Health Policy
University of Florida
Gainesville, FL

Lisa A. Schwartz, Ph.D.
The Children's Hospital of Philadelphia
Perelman School of Medicine, University of
Pennsylvania
Philadelphia, PA

Transition Care for Children With Special Health Needs

Structured Abstract

Background. Around 750,000 children in the United States with special health care needs transition to adult care annually. Fewer than half receive adequate support and services for their transition to adult care. Examples of programs with the potential to enhance transition for children with special heath care needs include use of a separate transition clinic, engagement of a transition coordinator, and a phased transfer within a clinical system. The potential for these programs to be effective is offset by barriers to their implementation.

Purpose. We developed a technical brief on the state of practice and the current literature around transition care for children with special health care needs to describe current practice and to provide a framework for future research.

Methods. We had conversations with Key Informants representing clinicians who provide transition care, pediatric and adult providers of services for individuals with special health care needs, policy experts, and researchers. We searched online sources for information about currently available programs and resources. We conducted a literature search to identify currently available research on the effectiveness of focused transition programs.

Findings. The issue of how to provide good transition care for children with special health care needs warrants further attention. The numbers of children with special health care needs reaching adulthood are increasing, and the diversity of their clinical conditions is expanding. The Got Transition resource provides a framework for transition care that can be adapted to serve the individual needs of a given patient population, but there is little evidence that it is used to provide a framework for evaluation in the research literature.

Despite identifying numerous descriptions of existing transition care programs or services, we identified only 25 evaluation studies, the majority of which did not include concurrent comparison groups. Most (n=8) were conducted in populations with diabetes, with a smaller literature (n=5) on transplant patients. We identified an additional 12 studies on a range of conditions, with no more than two studies on the same condition. Common components of care included use of a transition coordinator, a special clinic for young adults in transition and provision of educational materials, sometimes using computer-based programming.

An important consideration going forward is recognizing that transition care for chronic conditions like diabetes may warrant a different approach than care provided for more heterogeneous and complex conditions, particularly those that include a behavioral or intellectual component. Care for some patients may be appropriately provided in primary care at the community level; for others, it may be appropriately provided only in highly specialized regional or academic centers. Research needs are wide ranging, including both substantive and methodologic concerns. Currently, the field lacks a consistent and accepted way of measuring transition success, and it will be essential to establish consistent goals in order to build an adequate body of literature to affect practice.

Contents

Appendixes

Background

There is no uniformly accepted age at which pediatric care is inappropriate and adult care should be sought for every patient. Nonetheless, some practices do have age cut-offs, and there comes a time when adult providers may be better able to serve the needs of patients whose medical concerns are more adult in nature, including for example reproductive and other issues. In addition, the inclusion of adults in pediatric practices can create discomfort and challenges for other pediatric patients and their families, and pediatricians can find themselves addressing medical issues of adults for which they are less prepared. Therefore, at some point, most pediatric patients should and do move into the adult care system.

An effective transition process from a pediatric to an adult health system should ensure continuity of developmental and age-appropriate care. In 2002 the American Academy of Pediatrics (AAP), the American Academy of Family Physicians (AAFP), and the American College of Physicians (ACP) coauthored a consensus statement: "The goal of transition in health care for young adults with special health care needs is to maximize lifelong functioning and potential through the provision of high-quality, developmentally appropriate health care services that continue uninterrupted as the individual moves from adolescence to adulthood."[1]

This process can be challenging, particularly for children and youth with special health care needs (CSHCN), defined as individuals having or being at risk of "a chronic physical, developmental, behavioral, or emotional condition and who also require health and related services of a type or amount beyond that required by children generally."[2] Examples of adolescent populations with special health care needs that need transition support range widely, including those with chronic illnesses such as diabetes or sickle cell disease and individuals with developmental disabilities that are associated with a host of challenges ranging from higher risks of specific health outcomes to the need for special support in navigating the health care system.

The National Alliance to Advance Adolescent Health estimates that chronic health conditions affect approximately 25 percent of the 18 million U.S. young adults ages 18 to 21 who should be transitioning to adult-centered health care. Each year, approximately 750,000 young people in the United States with special health care needs transition to adult care.[3,4] Although they only represent an estimated 15.1 percent (2009/2010 National Survey of Children with Special Health Care Needs) to 19.8 percent (2011/2012 National Survey of Children's Health) of children aged 0 to 17 years, CSHCN account for as much as 70 percent of child health care expenditures,[5-7] and most of these individuals will survive into adulthood as the life expectancy of children with chronic illness continues to increase.[8,9] Over the past few decades, the prevalence of childhood chronic conditions also has been steadily increasing, with an associated increased risk of a range of health problems and persistent impact into adulthood for many affected individuals.[10,11]

Fewer than half of CSHCN aged 12 to 17 years report that they receive adequate support and services for their transition to adult care.[12-15] The proportion is even lower for ethnic minorities and children living in poverty,[16,17] with gaps in appropriate transitions to adult care ranging from approximately 15 to 25 percent.[17,18] The low rates of transition support reported by families may reflect the fact that only one-third of pediatricians report making referrals to adult physicians and less than 15 percent report providing transition education materials to adolescents and their parents.[19]

Potentially serious health-related consequences may be associated with suboptimal or incomplete transition to adult care. Gaps in care in transitions have been associated with poor health outcomes, increased hospitalizations and more complications and failure to access care in populations with diabetes, arthritis, and sickle cell disease.[20-24]

Examples of programs to enhance transition for CSHCN include use of a separate transition clinic, engagement of a transition coordinator, and a phased transfer within a clinical system.[20,25-27] The potential for these programs to be effective is offset by barriers that include a lack of time and resources to address transition issues, inadequate reimbursement, hesitancy of families and providers to dissolve long-standing therapeutic relationships, and gaps in residency training for both transition processes and medical management of adults with childhood-onset chronic diseases.[24,28-30] Additionally, CSHCN face broader challenges, including issues related to insurance, entitlements, guardianship, and eligibility for adult community-based services.[2,31]

Nonetheless, several guidelines, panels, and other groups coalesce around the need for good transition care for this population in particular. Healthy People 2010[32] includes a goal that all young people with special health care needs receive the services needed to make necessary transitions to all aspects of adult life, including health care. The AAP states that "optimal health care is achieved when every person at every age receives health care that is medically and developmentally appropriate."[1]

One of the six core objectives of the U.S. Department of Health and Human Services, Health Resources and Services Administration, Maternal and Child Health Bureau (MCHB) is that "all youth with special health care needs will receive the services necessary to make appropriate transitions to adult health care, work, and independence."[33] Despite this consistency in intent, there is little evidence to date about what constitutes an effective transition program for this population of patients,[34] although a literature of program descriptions, evaluations and research on the topic is growing.

The Affordable Care Act has several provisions reflecting federal emphasis on facilitating health care transitions for youth. Relevant provisions include extension of insurance for dependents and foster children up to age 26, protections that eliminate preexisting condition exclusions and lifetime coverage limits, Medicaid expansion, and creation of a new Center for Medicare and Medicaid Innovation that will include development and evaluation of patient-centered medical home models for individuals with complex needs.[35]

In 2011, the AAP, AAFP, and ACP[36] reaffirmed the 2002 jointly published consensus statement[1] and made further recommendations using a decision algorithm. The 2011 report describes practice-based recommendations and core elements, or components, of health care transition: transition policy, transitioning youth registry, transition preparation, transition planning, transition and transfer of care, and transition completion.[36] The components underscore the key concept that transition care is a process that involves actionable steps by both pediatric and adult provider. Transition is not a single event or passive process and the recommendations differentiate between health care transition and provider transfer, noting that, "[h]ealth care transfer is an element of transition and has a defined end point that may vary from patient to patient."[36]

Six common elements of transition planning that occur in both pediatric and adult practice are policy, patient registry, preparation, planning, transfer, and completion;[37] these are summarized in Got Transition,[38] a federally funded initiative. This initiative is a widely known resource to aid in transition planning and process, and when asked about standard components of transition planning, the Key Informants on this project consistently pointed to this approach. Importantly, the initiative describes standard elements for inclusion, but allows for the elements to be designed and implemented in a targeted manner to match the specific needs of the clinical condition or health care system. Thus, while the standard underlying elements are consistent, they are deployed in a targeted and specific manner. We elected to use these elements as a framework for organizing this literature.

A transition policy serves to educate staff about best practices for health care transition, with privacy and consent procedures shared with providers, staff, patients, and families. A patient registry is recommended for transition planning and monitoring outcomes. The Transition Readiness Assessment helps prepare patients for transition and identify gaps in knowledge or skills that may present educational opportunities for improvement in self-management. The Health Care Transition (HCT) Action Plans, including Portable Medical Summary and Emergency Care Plan are recommended for the planning phase. The Transfer of Care Checklist is also a useful tool for clinicians during the transfer of care phase. Finally, the pediatric care provider and team should follow up with the adult care team three months after transfer of care to ensure successful completion.[37]

Notable initiatives that make use of these six components include the National Health Care Transition Center multi-site learning collaborative, which piloted the six core elements of transition, and the Center for Medical Home Transition which includes visits from nurse case manager and sharing of information.[20] The National Health Care Transition Center also developed an assessment tool for use in the empirical evaluation of transition programs.[20,37]

Nonetheless, the currently available body of literature is primarily descriptive with only few studies that measure the effectiveness of any particular transition interventions, including use of the Got Transition framework. Much of the research emphasizes the transfer component of transition, and completion of transfer is a common outcome. Although we attempted to review the state of the literate on the complete transition process, the availability of literature across elements was clearly not consistent and that is reflected in our results.

Technical Brief Objectives

Despite a lack of rigorous research on the topic, various organizations have suggested that transition planning is particularly important for children and adolescents with special health care needs. Descriptive studies have been published and the empirical literature is growing, but the study data needed to conduct a meaningful systematic review of transition effectiveness either is not yet available or has not been published. We therefore developed a Technical Brief to report existing programs or approaches for transition care and describe the current state of the research.

A Technical Brief is a rapid report of an emerging intervention for which there are limited published data and too few completed research studies to support definitive conclusions. The goals of the Technical Brief are to provide an objective description of the state of the science, identify a potential framework for assessing the applications and implications of the intervention, summarize ongoing research, and present research gaps. A technical brief is not intended to be a comprehensive systematic review but should provide the reader with an overview of available research, practice and to some degree, perspective, around a given clinical intervention.

For this Technical Brief, we proposed Guiding Questions to summarize the purpose and components of transition care for CSHCNs, describe the clinical practice areas that evaluated strategies for transition care, outline possible training and barriers to transition care, and identify directions for future research. We outlined the report scope and priorities with input from Key Informants identified as individuals who were engaged in the practice, implementation, or evaluation of existing programs and systems of transition care for youth with special health needs.

This report focuses specifically on transitions of care from pediatric to adult services for individuals with a chronic health condition. It does not include transitions within the adult health care system or the transition of youth without a special health care need. Similarly, we confined the scope of the proposed Guiding Questions to transition in health care, with the understanding that the provision of clinical services is a part of a comprehensive evaluation of successful transition that would likely include educational, psychosocial, and occupational supports.

Guiding Questions

We presented the following questions to the Key Informants:

Guiding Question 1. Description of Interventions for Transition Care

a. What are the goals of transition care and what are the theoretical advantages and disadvantages?
b. What are the common components of transition care interventions or processes used in clinical practice for children/adolescents with special health care needs?
c. How do currently used approaches to transitioning health care address the complexity of health issues including comorbidities and the presence of both physical and intellectual/developmental disabilities?

Guiding Question 2. Description of the Context for Implementing Transition Care

a. How widely available are programs or approaches to transition care within the health care setting for children/adolescents with special health care needs?
b. What are the resources needed to implement transition care?
c. What are the specific barriers to implementing transition care or processes for children/adolescents with special health care needs?
d. Who delivers transition interventions and what training is required to implement identified approaches to transition care for children/adolescents with special health care needs?

Guiding Question 3. Description of the Existing Evidence

a. What patient groups/clinical conditions are represented in studies on the use and evaluation of transition care for children/adolescents with special health care needs?
b. What is the length of followup in studies on the use and evaluation of transition care for children/adolescents with special health care needs?
c. What outcomes are measured in studies on the use and evaluation of transition care for children/adolescents with special health care needs?

Guiding Question 4. Issues and Future Research

a. What are the implications (e.g., ethical, privacy, economic) of the current level of diffusion and of further diffusion of transition care for children/adolescents with special health care needs?

b. What are possible areas of future research for transition care for children/adolescents with special health care needs and which research designs are most appropriate to address these research topics?

Methods

We used discussions with Key Informants, a search of the gray literature, and a search of the published literature to collect relevant data and descriptions.

Data Collection

Discussions With Key Informants

We engaged Key Informants to offer insight into the clinical context of transition care, and suggest issues of greatest importance to clinicians, patients, researchers, and payers. We searched the Web sites of relevant professional organizations and research and policy groups to identify stakeholders whose work or interests indicate a high likelihood of interest and expertise in the topic.

In consultation with the investigative team and the Agency for Healthcare Research and Quality (AHRQ), we assembled a list of individuals representing a clinical, policy, research, or advocate perspective for transition care. Four of 18 invited individuals agreed to participate. Following approval by AHRQ of the completed Disclosure of Interest forms for proposed Key Informants, we conducted discussions with four Key Informants, representing clinicians in practice as well as in policy roles in addition to accomplished researchers.

We conducted one group discussion by telephone with Key Informants. We invited the Key Informants to share their experiences and make suggestions to the proposed Technical Brief. Before the call, we developed a list of general guiding questions for call participants and provided the call participants with a copy of the proposed guiding questions. We asked Key Informants to provide perspective on the CSHCN populations and clinical subgroups of interest, interventions for comparison, relevant outcomes, timing for interventions and outcomes, and other information that would make this report most useful to decision makers. We recorded and transcribed the call discussion and generated a summary that we distributed to call participants.

We used the input from the Key Informants to confirm our initial findings and verify the feasibility of the scope established by the team for the Technical Brief. In particular, we asked Key Informants about issues related to definitions, clinical areas, population, implementation, resources, and future research needs.

Published Literature Search

We used a combination of controlled vocabulary terms and keywords to search the published literature for studies that specifically evaluated transition programs. The definition of CSHCN is broad and may encompass many diagnoses and substantial heterogeneity in medical complexity. We used a terms for specific chronic diseases (e.g., asthma) and disabilities (e.g., blindness), as well as broad terms (e.g., congenital defects) and descriptors of youth with special health needs and transition care (e.g., continuity of patient care). We searched the literature base from 2000 on. We reviewed the reference lists of retrieved publications for other potentially relevant publications missed by the search strategies. We present the literature search details in Appendix A.

To identify newly published relevant literature, we updated the literature search during peer review and the posting period for public comments. We incorporated the results from the literature update into the Technical Brief.

We developed forms (Appendix B) for screening and data collection from the published literature. We recorded the study design and study populations from relevant sources. We focused on transition care from pediatric to adult services for individuals with chronic conditions. We did not limit by clinical condition, as a goal of this review was to identify common characteristics of effective transition support across clinical conditions. We limited by type of care, excluding studies of transition care in the context of palliative or hospice care.

We further limited the literature search results for Guiding Question 3 to original research studies. Table 1 summarizes the inclusion and exclusion criteria for the evaluation studies that were included in Guiding Question 3. We scanned the text of all included publications for information on barriers, training needs, variation in practice, and the potential impact of transition care on economic and policy decisions.

Table 1. Inclusion and exclusion criteria for evaluation studies

Category	Criteria
Study population	Children with special health care needs
Publication languages	English only

Admissible evidence (study design and other criteria)	Admissible designs
	Randomized controlled trials(including wait-list control), cohorts with comparison, pre-post cohort without comparison, stepped wedge designs, case-control, case series, and case reports
	Other criteria
	• Original research studies that provide sufficient detail regarding methods and results to enable use and adjustment of the data and results.
	• Studies must address the following for transitions in care:
	   ○ Transitions of care from pediatric to adult services.
	   ○ Children with special health needs as defined by the American Academy of Pediatrics.
	   ○ A special health need that arises from a chronic physical, developmental, or intellectual condition or disability.

Gray Literature Search

We augmented the searches we conducted in bibliographic databases by searching for gray literature. Examples of sources of gray literature include the Internet, government Web sites, clinical trial databases, trade publications, and meeting abstracts. We crosschecked the findings from the gray literature searches against the literature retrieval for publications that we may have missed in the literature searches.

We searched Web sites of relevant professional associations and patient advocate groups for information on transition care programs and strategies for special health care needs. We performed searches of public health department Web sites for each state for online descriptions or links to existing transition care programs or models. We accessed NIH RePORTER, HSRProj, and ClinicalTrials.gov to identify ongoing research. Appendix C presents details of our findings from the gray literature.

Data Organization and Presentation

We summarize information extracted from the published and gray literature in the results and discussion of this report. We organize the transition care components into categories and describe commonalities among existing transition care models or programs, as well as approaches that warrant further evaluation (Guiding Question 1). We identify resources for and barriers to adoption and implementation of transition care (Guiding Question 2). We present information on current practice and research in summary tables and text (Guiding Question 3). We highlight the implications of existing transition care practice and the need for future research in Guiding Question 4.

We used gray literature sources to locate innovative transition care models and programs and present this information in tables in Appendix C. We catalogued information on transition care services from individual States and health care systems as it was available (Appendix C). We documented reasons for exclusion of records that were promoted for full text review (Appendix D).

Peer Review

A draft of this Technical Brief was posted to the AHRQ Web site for 4 weeks for public comments. During this time, the Scientific Resource Center distributed the draft report to individuals who agreed to serve as peer reviewers. The Scientific Resource Center collected the feedback from peer reviewers and forwarded the compiled comments to report authors. We reviewed the comments and made appropriate changes to the final report.

We documented the report revisions and provided a summary of responses to the individual comments received from public and peer reviewers in a disposition of comments table. The disposition of comments table will be available on the AHRQ Web site after publication of the final Technical Brief Report.

Findings

In this section, we summarize information from the published and gray literature sources to address Guiding Questions 1–4. Much of the discussion with Key Informants was consistent with the salient topics that emerged from the body of literature, focusing primarily upon the need for, implications of, and barriers to the adoption of seamless, effective, and comprehensive transition care for children and youth with special health care needs (CSHCN).

We summarize the literature on the purpose and current approaches for transition care using the framework of Got Transition[38] as an organizational structure (Guiding Question 1). This is not an endorsement of the framework, but as the most well-known and publicly available approach, it provides a logical and accessible organizational structure. We then provide a discussion of resources, barriers and other contextual issues important to the implementation and adoption of transition strategies (Guiding Question 2). The results presented here are a combination of a summary of the literature and our Key Informant conversations. We present the state of the current research, identifying the sources and findings from evaluation studies of transition approaches in Guiding Question 3. We present implications and areas for future research in Guiding Question 4.

Guiding Question 1. Description of Interventions for Transition Care

a. What are the goals of transition care and what are the theoretical advantages and disadvantages?
b. What are the common components of transition care interventions or processes used in clinical practice for children/adolescents with special health care needs?
c. How do currently used approaches to transitioning health care address the complexity of health issues including comorbidities and the presence of both physical and intellectual/developmental disabilities?

Goals of Transition Care (Guiding Question1a)

The provision of high quality transition care for youth with special health care needs should optimize the patient's quality of life and ensure continued access to and appropriate use of clinical care.[34,36,39-46] More specifically, the American Academy of Pediatrics (AAP) suggests that good transition care follow the principles of the medical home. Transition care should be coordinated, comprehensive, individualized, culturally competent, and patient-centered.[27,40,43,47-57] The AAP also recommends that the transition program promote skills in communication, decision-making, assertiveness, and self-care to enhance a sense of control and independence of health care for youth.[40,43,55]

Several professional organizations including the American Academy of Family Physicians (AAFP), the American College of Physicians (ACP), the Society for Adolescent Health and Medicine, the Canadian Pediatric Society, and the National Association of Pediatric Nurse Practitioners and Nurses also endorse these functional goals.[50,58-60] Key Informants in this process stated that transition care should be based upon these principles, but that specific programs should be designed to match the specific needs of the patient population and the health care system.

Increased prevalence of chronic and disabling disease paired with improvements in early diagnosis and treatment of those conditions have led to increasing numbers of children and youth with special health care needs living into adulthood.[27,34,61-65] Based on the most recent estimate from the AAP in 2002, more than 90 percent of CSHCN now survive into adulthood, and approximately 750,000 CSHCN make the transition to adulthood annually in the United States.[1,34,51,58,60,66-70]

Current practice involves a range from simple transfer of care from pediatric to adult settings that occurs at a set time-point to a well-planned and coordinated transition of care that occurs over time and encompasses elements both before and after the anticipated transfer of care.[71-73] When transition involves only an abrupt care transfer, patients may be put at risk of getting "lost in the system" or experiencing decreased access to care, both of which may be associated with poorer long-term health outcomes, impaired function, and high-cost emergency care.[49,50,65,67,74,75] One of the goals of transition care is therefore to prevent these adverse outcomes.

Advantages

Proposed benefits of purposeful transition care are that it provides youth with ongoing access to primary care and subspecialist care, promotes competence in disease management, fosters independence, social, and emotional development through teaching self-advocacy and communication skills, and allows for a sense of security for support of long-term health care planning and life goals. Self-care behaviors learned from well-executed health transition care during adolescence may also be useful during other periods of transition, such as changes in residence, insurance, and personal preference.[76]

Direct benefits of transition care to the patient include improved disease control, decreased hospital admissions, better quality of life, and increased patient satisfaction,[77-79] but further research is needed to determine how best to implement transition care and if such efforts translate into long-term improvements in overall health outcomes.[75,80] Transfer of care to an adult provider, as a component of transition care, provides the benefit of access to targeted care for issues related to adulthood and aging, which may be better handled by adult providers. Adult providers are also better suited to address issues such as pregnancy and comorbidities associated with adult lifestyle and aging.[81,82]

Finally, post-transition perspective surveys suggest that although CSHCN appreciate the increased autonomy received in adult clinics, they report that a transition program (as opposed to a transfer of care) would be beneficial.[83,84]

Disadvantages

An inherent disadvantage of transfer of care includes a change in the health care provider and a move away from a familiar pediatric setting. As illustrated in a study published in 2011 that assessed the transfer experiences and medical outcomes of a cohort of individuals with HIV acquired in childhood, the transition to adult care was more difficult than expected, and youth reported feelings of abandonment and sadness with the loss of patient-provider relationship after transfer to adult health care. Almost one half of the participants who transferred to adult care (19/42) reported problems with medication adherence. This study also reported that CD4 counts trended downward, clinically indicating worsening disease status, from pre- to post-transfer.[85] Other studies report young adults with sickle cell disease transferring from pediatric clinics experiencing increased episodes of pain and greater mortality,[86-88] premature deaths after transfer for young people with congenital heart disease,[63] and high rates of rejection and allograft loss among youth with transplants immediately following transfer.[42,63,81,89,90]

Some subgroups of patients may be at increased risk for poorer outcomes. For example, a retrospective review of administrative and survey data of young adults with diabetes found that individuals in the lowest income group were less likely to attend an eye care visit in the two years after transition to adult diabetes care than were individuals from other income groups.[23] Patients transferred to a new health care team who did not change physicians were less likely to be hospitalized after the transfer than were patients who changed physicians, regardless of whether or not they also transferred to a new health care team.[23]

None of these disadvantages is related to good transition planning; rather these are disadvantages of moving from a pediatric health care system to an adult health care system in circumstances where there are inadequate supports. Actual disadvantages of well-executed transition care have not been formally studied. At the system level, potential disadvantages of true transition care may include high costs of providing care and lack of reimbursement for these services, costs of system changes during development and implementation phases for transition programs, and loss of revenue for children's hospitals (i.e. movement of congenital heart disease cases to adult hospitals). However, studies comparing cost-effectiveness of transition care for children with special health care needs and cost of unsuccessful transition are lacking.

Components of Transition Care (Guiding Question 1b)

Although there is common endorsement in the literature for the need for transition planning for CSHCN, a range of approaches to improving the process and structure of transition care has been proposed, and no gold standard for transition care exists.[51,64,83,90] The most common practice models are: a primary care model where the general practitioner provides ongoing medical care and implements and/or uses transition related services and supports, a transition coordination model where a consultative, multidisciplinary team facilitates the transition, and an adolescent-focused model where youth transition to adult care through an adolescent specialist service.[45,70,91] Disease-specific or subspecialty-based transition programs also exist and may use any one of the models described above in a disease-specific way.[54,64,70,75,79,92-95]

It is worth noting that although patients cared for by family practitioners may theoretically have the same primary care physician in childhood and adulthood, these patients may still benefit from a process to help them assume increasing responsibility for their own care as they age and may still need to transfer some of their care from pediatric to adult specialists. There are no empirical data in the literature to guide decisions regarding whether primary care transition and subspecialty care transitions should occur simultaneously or in a sequential fashion.

Key informants noted that varying approaches to transition care may be warranted and appropriate given the heterogeneity of CSHCN, both by diagnosis and by level of medical complexity. For example, discussion of infection control policies will be an important aspect of transition programs for patients with cystic fibrosis,[96] while transition programs for youth with HIV will likely incorporate strategies to address the stigma surrounding this diagnosis.[57,77,83] The format that is adopted also depends on the facilities and resources available.[39,43,53,56,58,62,64,82,97-99] Likewise, the Society for Adolescent Medicine recommends that one of the basic principles for successful transition is "to have individualized and flexible enough programs to meet the needs of young people and their families."[68,75]

Despite documented variation and a focus on flexibility in transition approaches, there is a core set of common components of quality transition care. Experts, including this project's Key Informants, point to the Got Transition Six Core Elements of Health Care Transition[37] as a useful framework that is widely accessible and flexible. Got Transition is the name of The National

Alliance to Advance Adolescent Health initiative supported by the U.S. Maternal and Child Bureau/Health Resources and Services Administration. These efforts led four practice-based Breakthrough Series-style Learning Collaboratives, adapting quality improvement methodology used by the National Initiative for Children's Healthcare Quality (NICHQ) and pioneered by the Institute for Healthcare Improvement (IHI) to generate and test its suggested transition framework.

The core elements defined by Got Transition[38] mirror the algorithm for best practices in the clinical report titled "Supporting the Health Care Transition From Adolescence to Adulthood in the Medical Home" that was jointly published by the AAP, AAFP, and ACP.[36,37] These core elements, or components, of health care transition are transition policy, transitioning youth registry, transition preparation, transition planning, transition and transfer of care, and transition completion and apply to both pediatric and adult health care settings.[38] These components underscore the key concept that transition care is a process that involves actionable steps by both pediatric and adult provider, not a single event or passive process.

Each of these components can be augmented by the use of specific tools to address issues including comorbidities, the presence of both physical and intellectual disabilities, and confounding psychosocial circumstances. Different tools may be used for different groups of patients or different clinical settings. Incorporation and implementation of different tools also may vary based on available resources and support services. Most published transition programs incorporate multiple components and tools, making assessment of individual components difficult.[78,100]

We have organized the review of the literature addressing transition care components (Guiding Question 1b) around the Got Transition[38] algorithm based on advice from this project's Key Informants. However, given the recognized need for further evidence-based recommendations in this field, we do not formally endorse the program. Rather, as noted elsewhere in this report, we use it as an organizing tool; we recognize that some users of this report may prefer other approaches to organizing the literature.

Transition Policy

An explicit transition policy describes the practice's approach to health care transition, outlines goals of the program, and clarifies the roles and responsibilities of the youth, family, and health care team.[36,43,52,75,97,101-103] Development of policies may involve both pediatric and adult transition teams.[62,92,104,105]

The transition policy typically includes a timeline with a suggested age for beginning the transition process and tentative deadline for ultimate transfer of care.[40,97] It is frequently recommended in the published literature that transition care start early, perhaps as young as 10 to 12 years of age, to allow for an adequate period of preparation,[43,52,53,60,62,66,74,83,97,99,105-111] and some advocate for beginning the process at time of diagnosis.[112,113] There is little empirical evidence, however, about optimal age at which to begin the process.

Timing of transfer takes into account the youth's cognitive development, physical abilities, and environment, which includes socioeconomic characteristics and psychosocial resources including family or peer support.[48,51,57,99,109,112,114-116] In particular, it is typically recommended that transfer of care not take place during a period of health crisis, especially if the support system is unstable.[99,113,115-118]

Nonetheless, having a target age of transfer could be useful to catalyze transition activities to plan and prepare for the ultimate transfer of care. Age 18 years is most commonly considered an acceptable age for transfer,[62,65,92,106,112,114,119] and this is the age at which parents loose access to their child's medical records. However, the range of suggested age of transfer is from 12 years[100] to 25 years.[97,120] The wide range of suggested transfer age in the literature may underscore that timing of transfer of care should be individualized.[100,120,121]

Other suggestions for introducing anticipated transition that we identified in our search were transition alert letters, videos, and pamphlets or books.[61,122] Pamphlets, in particular, theoretically offer an accessible, portable, convenient, and cost-effective means for information distribution.[122]

Transition Registry

Some medical practices maintain transition registries to help identify patients with special health care needs at the appropriate chronologic age for transition and enable a system for monitoring which steps of the transition process still need to be completed.[36,97] Use of electronic health record systems can facilitate development and organization of such registries.[123] Minimal information is available at this time regarding the utility of and implementation strategies for transition registries as a component of a transition program. Nonetheless, the use of a registry to track the status of patients with special health care needs and also to stratify them in terms of complexity is endorsed as an important distinction of a medical home.[36]

Transition Preparation

Youth, their families and their providers all need to be prepared to initiate and complete a transition process. Key Informants reported that providers may not have access to adequate training to manage the challenges associated with transition and that adult providers may be unprepared to care for CSHCN who transfer to adult care, and this opinion is echoed the published literature. Thus, transition care involves active preparation on the part of providers, transitioning youth, and their families. Educational needs exist for both the clinical team and the patients and their families in preparation for transition.[34,40,66,111,117]

First, some health care providers may need additional education on transition care topics and professional training in caring for adolescent patients.[36,66,103,124] Team members may need to be supported with continuing medical education programs that are tailored for their specific functional needs as a member of the transition team.[87] One specific educational resource for health care providers is the Transition-Oriented Health Supervision (TOHS), based upon the American Academy of Pediatrics Bright Futures developmental approach to health supervision, which helps guide clinical encounters to prepare CSHCN, and their families, for the necessary move from pediatric to adult health care.[19] The AAP is also developing Maintenance of Certification modules addressing transition planning.[123]

Second, youth and family report a need for education about the differences between pediatric and adult care and may receive ongoing anticipatory guidance regarding what to expect from adult specialty care[36,66,83,118] as well as instruction for navigating the system of entitlements, such as Medicaid and Supplemental Security Income.[55,83] Youth and their parents also report the need for disease-specific education during this time.[125]

Transition should include a formal transition curriculum to address medical and non-medical issues including disease-specific topics, skills training in communication, decisionmaking, creative problem solving, assertiveness, self-care, self-determination, and self-advocacy.[43,51-53,57,66,71,75,78,103,116] Incorporation of online materials and text messaging can be a useful tool to promote health management skills in adolescents.[126]

Transition preparation also is recommended to include support for youth and their family.[43,51,55,60,82,98,101,111,117] Both family and peer support groups or mentoring programs have been proposed as forms of support and education during the transition process.[36,54,77,97,99,108-110,112,126,127] The Adolescent Leadership Council[128] is an example of a group-mentoring program that brings together high school students with chronic illness and college student mentors with chronic illness. Participants have reported that they learned to better care for their illness and gained skills talking about their illness, and investigators reported a small increase in transition readiness scores for participants in the program, although successful transitioning has not been evaluated.[128]

Another example is the Good2Go Transition Program[129] which used psycho-educational transition groups to discuss issues of self-advocacy, independent behaviors, health lifestyle issues, and health care access strategies. These groups were also available to support parents in growing independence of their adolescent.[50]

Mentoring via email or internet chat rooms has also been proposed but not evaluated.[54,130] Summer camps are another option that could provide opportunities to increase social networks and promote development of self-management skills.[131]

Transition care programs typically attempt to be family-centered and engage the family in the process by recognizing that the family's role in care of the young adult is not necessarily diminishing, but changing to a more consultative role for health care needs.[43,54,83,99,107,132]

Some studies report that continued involvement of parents in youth's lives has a protective effect on better health outcomes.[125,133] Thus, transition planning with parents may be a beneficial aspect of transition preparation for the youth.[75,134] Examples of opportunities for family engagement include concurrent visits for parents, specific focus on fathers, and modeling of healthy lifestyles.[42,44,78,101,135] Printed materials to educate and coach parents about their evolving role, particularly as it pertains to communication and co-management, are available through Family Voices.[136]

Transition Planning

Individualized Transition Plan

There is a marked emphasis in the literature supporting a formal, individualized transition plan documented in the medical record.[1,34,36,42,43,52,57,65,97,99,101,112,137,138] Careful documentation in the patient chart of intent to transfer to an adult health care provider and details regarding transition conversations among patients and providers may predict successful transfer of care.[76,107] The transition plan generally includes goals for achieving self-care, health care decision-making, and self-advocacy and outlines specific actions required to achieve these goals.[60,67] The transition plan also documents the expectations for the adolescent's knowledge and understanding about his or her condition[57,66] and addresses strategies for securing health insurance.[34] Key informants provided information on the degree to which developing such a plan is time intensive, but essential for ensuring that the process goes well.

In theory, collaborative development of a transition plan may enhance communication between the patient and the health care provider and helps parents learn to consider their child's future capacity in multiple domains such as education, employment, and independent living, and it helps adolescents learn that they will be expected to take gradual increased responsibility for their health care.[76,139] Enhancing patient-provider communication has been cited as a means for smoothing the transition to adult care.[140] Multiple approaches may be used to facilitate

14

communication; for example holding visits in a consultation room without examination equipment and the provider-patient dialogue taking place sitting around a table rather than behind a desk.[141]

Assessing Readiness

Most transition programs suggest that assessment of transition readiness can guide individualized interventions that promote appropriate patient education and skill development.[36,49,66,97,98,108,122] Readiness assessment tools also offer the added advantage of measuring overlapping constructs or assessing the continuum of transition preparedness as opposed to the simple "yes/no" questions on checklists.[49,67,98] Readiness assessment tools can also be used to measure clinical outcomes of developing transition programs.[142] A systematic review completed by Stinson and colleagues in September 2012 identified seven transition readiness measures, but found that none of these tools had been appropriately psychometrically tested to establish validity and reliability.[142]

In the absence of rigorously tested transition readiness tools, use of behavior theories, such as the transtheoretical model and stages of change, to assess patient readiness has been suggested. The five stages of change in the transtheoretical model are precontemplation, contemplation, preparation, action, and maintenance and can describe transition from a patient who has not yet considered transition to the adult health care system through a patient that fully accepts responsibility for his/her health.[102]

Legal Considerations

Some youth with special health care needs will not attain independence because of significant developmental or functional disabilities. Discussions about guardianship, health care power of attorney, and other legal issues may need to take place during transition preparation.[36,123,143] It is recommended that such youth have a functional competency assessment well before age 18 to determine specific supports needed and arrange for these supports in order to increase self-determination.[111]

Medical providers providing transition care recognize that parents appointed as legal guardians will remain involved in the youth's care for the remainder of the individual's life.[51] Appropriate steps can be taken to ensure these parents continue to have access to their child's medical records even after their child reaches 18 years of age. Parental estate planning to protect Supplemental Security Income eligibility should also be considered during the transition planning period.[111] The transition period also provides an opportunity to hold end-of-life and emergency planning discussions collaboratively and without urgency.[53,116,143]

Transfer of Care

The transfer of care from a pediatric to adult provider is just one concrete aspect of the overall transition process. Nonetheless, much of the empirical literature uses successful transfer as a measure of effectiveness.

Checklists, portable medical summaries, and meeting the adult provider before transfer are often recommended as part of the transfer of care process.[48,62,63,96,98,99,102,103,109,114,135,144] Table 2 summarizes specific examples of these tools.

Table 2. Tools to aid transition and transfer

Tool	Description	Examples
Checklists	<ul><li>May be placed in the patients' charts</li><li>Allows providers to keep track of the skills and knowledge that the transitioning youth needs to acquire before transfer of care</li><li>May be used to ensure that all crucial education topics are covered</li><li>May divide tasks based on chronological age</li><li>Clinical decision support systems that remind clinical teams about steps for transition planning</li></ul>	<ul><li>Spina Bifida Transition Program at the University of Wisconsin[82]</li><li>Clinical Pathway Document developed by the ON TRAC program at British Columbia Children's Hospital[145]</li><li>Checklist developed at the Center for Inflammatory Bowel Disease at Children's Hospital Boston[146]</li><li>Rheumatology transition program at the Princess of Wales Children's Hospital, Birmingham, United Kingdom[101]</li><li>Checklist available through the Endocrine Society's online practice management resource [79]</li></ul>
Portable Medical Summary	<ul><li>May include past medical and surgical history, list of current medications, allergies, immunizations, pertinent family and social history, most recent diagnostic and imaging studies, disease specific parameters (i.e., cardiac anatomy and physiology for patients with congenital heart disease), upcoming appointments, and contact information for health care providers</li><li>Updated at each visit and a copy should be included in the medical record and given to the adolescent to keep</li><li>May require special adaptation for those with intellectual disability to include non-written forms of communication such as pictures or tape recordings</li></ul>	<ul><li>*MyHealth Passport* developed by the *Good2Go* Transition Program at the Hospital for Sick Children[129,147]</li><li>*Your Plan It* developed by the ON TRAC program at the British Columbia Children's Hospital[145]</li></ul>
Meeting the Adult Provider	<ul><li>May alleviate the lack of trust, fear, and anxiety that the youth and family may have related to acquiring a new adult provider</li><li>May increase confidence and comfort among transitioning youth</li><li>May promote higher rates of retention in adult clinics after transfer</li><li>Joint clinics (or appointments) are a strategy for patients to meet the adult provider(s) before the transfer of care and help facilitate communication and convey trust among pediatric and adult members of the transition team</li><li>Tours of receiving adult clinics are another strategy used to enable patients to meet the accepting adult health care team before transfer and acclimate the patient to their new health care setting</li></ul>	<ul><li>Spina Bifida Transition Program at the University of Wisconsin[82]</li><li>Cystic Fibrosis Transition Program at the University of Michigan[148]</li><li>Young Persons Clinic at the Royal Manchester Children's Hospital[149]</li><li>University Diabetes Center in Italy[150]</li><li>Transition Pilot Program at St. Jude Children's Hospital[148]</li><li>Sickle Cell Transition Program at Froedtert Hospital and Medical College of Wisconsin, Milwaukee[151]</li><li>MAGICC approach in the Rheumatology Divisions at the Royal Hallamshire Hospital and Sheffield Children's Hospital[105]</li><li>Royal Gwent Hospital diabetes program,[120] Newport</li><li>DON'T RETARD transition program for youth with juvenile idiopathic arthritis at University Hospitals Leuven, Belgium[78]</li><li>The Liverpool Model, Liverpool Heart and Chest Hospital, United Kingdom[121]</li></ul>

16

Transition Completion

Written communication and good documentation may serve to promote continuity of care.[36,48,66,68,83,97,104,130,152] Maintaining an up to date medical summary that is portable and accessible enables such communication.[1,42,106,110,113,116] The medical summary for transition includes recommendations for treatments that work best physiologically and psychologically for the individual patient and family, as well as details such as advanced directives and provisions for affordable, continuous health insurance coverage.[53,57,65,79,116,122] Providing the patient with a copy of the portable medical summary may help with communication and allows the patient an opportunity to include any personal information and advanced directives that he chooses.[50,63,75,97,108] Personally controlled electronic health records or emerging smart phone applications can help support this effort.[123] It may be helpful to have youth prepare their own referral letter to clarify their medical needs and set objectives for self-management, promoting identity development and responsibility.[119]

It is typically recommended that the referring pediatric team be available to the adult team as a resource immediately after the transfer of care to allow for a period of co-management with pediatric and adult providers.[97,113] A transition coordinator, specifically, can help bridge communication between the pediatric and adult teams upon completing transfer of care.[66,97] Some programs have included a celebration, including certificates, letters of gratitude to the health team, and graduation ceremonies.[72,106,110,137,153] These strategies may address the feelings of abandonment and sadness with the loss of patient-provider relationship that youth have reported after transfer to adult health care.[23]

After complete transfer of care has taken place, the overall transition process should be evaluated to highlight areas for future improvement.[54,97,103-105,112,117] Participation of youth and their families in evaluation of transition care also is recommended when developing and improving transition services.[110] Continual transition service improvement will require the development more robust data collection methods and measurement tools that reflect the essential components of transition.[134,154]

Such tools could be developed in conjunction with electronic clinical decision support systems that aid health care providers in completing the sequential steps of transition planning, particularly since decision support and clinical information systems are two of the six "pillars" of the Care Model for Child Health.[155] The systematic review conducted by Stinson and colleagues in September 2012 identified six transfer satisfaction measures, but found that none of these tools had well-established evidence of reliability and validity and most did not comment on how CSHCN or their families had been involved in the development and testing of these patient-reported outcome measures.[142]

Transition in the Face of Patient Complexity (Guiding Question 1c)

Youth with special health care needs often have a complex array of medical and sometimes psychological or psychiatric conditions, reinforcing the need for individualized transition care. Each of the general components above can be personalized or augmented by the use of specific tools to address the complexity of health issues including comorbidities, the presence of both physical and intellectual disabilities, and confounding psychosocial circumstances.

The following may be helpful for addressing complexity in patient populations: maintaining a flexible policy regarding the timing of the transfer, adequate preparation through focused education and support, development of individualized transition plans, utilization of a transition coordinator, and facilitated communication between multidisciplinary providers and patient or family through use of a portable medical summary.

Our Key Informants noted that while all adolescents with a chronic condition would need some sort of transition support. Furthermore, their diversity in terms of conditions and complexity affects what is needed and where. For highly complex cases, the range and quantity of resources may be available, for example, only at centralized programs, often at academic centers. For some types of chronic conditions, on the other hand, and in the absence of multiple conditions, Key Informants recommended that community based programs can and should be developed.

Guiding Question 2. Description of the Context for Implementing Transition Care

a. How widely available are programs or approaches to transition care within the health care setting for children/adolescents with special health care needs?
b. What are the resources needed to implement transition care?
c. What are the specific barriers to implementing transition care or processes for children/adolescents with special health care needs?
d. Who delivers transition interventions and what training is required to implement identified approaches to transition care for children/adolescents with special health care needs?

Availability of Transition Programs (Guiding Question 2a)

The data on availability of transition programs are limited, but the little research that has been done suggests that these programs are not widely available. Although current numbers are unavailable, about one-half of diabetes centers in the United States reported having a structured transition program in 2010,[156] and only 18 percent of pediatric rheumatology units in the United Kingdom had a dedicated adolescent clinic in 2000.[40]

Transition services might be especially inaccessible if one is receiving public services in childhood;[65] a survey of state mental health administrators from across the United States found that only 5 percent reported the existence of any type of programs or services within the State mental health system to transition mental health treatment from the child to adult service system.[157] Thus, the findings from limited research converge around some level of inaccessibility of transition programs and services, with anywhere from 5 to 50 percent of agencies or clinics offering such programs. Key Informants affirmed that availability and resources rather than standards defined as best practice and resources shape the landscape of transition care approaches seen in practice.

Dedicated transition programs are not only relatively inaccessible, but many pediatric clinics do not have formal plans for transitioning their pediatric patients with special health care needs to adult care. In a survey of providers of pediatric HIV care in the United States, 81 percent had designated a transition coordinator, but few clinics had established policies to define the details of transition.[14] Established transition policies were also relatively uncommon in a survey of primary care pediatricians in the United States; only 13 percent had written policies about the transition from pediatric to adult care.[158]

Aside from information on the availability of specific transition programs or plans, the proportion of youth with special health care needs who are given information and assistance with transition (either within the context of a transition program or through their pediatric provider) is low. Nationally, only about 40 percent of youth with special health care needs meet criteria for adequate transition support, with the other 60 percent being unprepared for transition in at least one area.[14,159] Similarly, among young adults with diabetes only 50 percent reported receiving specific adult provider or clinic recommendations. Fewer than 15 percent of participants reported receiving written transition materials, having a specific visit to discuss transition, or meeting the adult provider before transition.[160] Finally, less than 40 percent of a sample of young adults with sickle cell disease received any preparation before transferring from pediatric to adult care.[161]

Perhaps in part because of a lack of transition support, just over 20 percent of youth with special health care needs nationally have successfully transitioned to adult care, defined by constructs such as having an adult provider who provides routine preventative care and having continuous health insurance coverage.[162]

In sum, the limited data on the availability of transition programs and information suggests that the majority of transitioning youth with special health care needs do not have access to a specific program to aid with their transition, nor to the necessary information or planning to make the transition a smooth process. Lack of access appears to be particularly pronounced for youth who are not receiving care within a medical home setting[13] or are receiving public assistance, as well as youth with certain neurodevelopmental or psychiatric conditions,[163] whose parents have less education, and who are racial/ethnic minorities.[17,162]

Our search for transition programs with information available online identified specific programs, presented in Appendix C. Few of these programs are evaluated in the published or gray literature. The gray literature search also retrieved a variety of online resources for transition care for individuals with special health needs.

Resources To Implement Transition Care (Guiding Question 2b)

The resources needed to implement transition care vary, of course, by the type or complexity of the program or service. Commonly described resources include space, time, personnel, materials, and systems for knowledge transfer. Key Informants noted that successful implementation of a transition care program requires significant staffing and resources.

Space

Like all other health care programs, transition programs require dedicated space. Some transition programs use space to create a dedicated transition clinic.[71,149,164-167] In other transition programs, space is needed to house a dedicated transition coordinator or other personnel within a pediatric clinic. Still other transition programs require space to convene transition-related activities such as peer support or mentoring groups.[128,168]

Time

Time is necessary to develop and implement transition policies, establish and maintain transition registries, prepare patients and families for transition, and transition planning and actual case transfer. For example, transition preparation, planning and case transfer all require communication and coordination between pediatric and adult providers.[62,64,82,139,169-171] This requires patients and their families, pediatric providers, and adult providers to dedicate time to these activities.

It may be particularly important for adult providers to allow additional time for the first post-transition appointment because this may help build rapport with transitioning youth and their family and help the provider understand the youth's health care needs.[82] Flexibility in terms of when the first adult appointment is scheduled may also be helpful. For example, scheduling the first adult provider appointment close in time to the last pediatric appointment, instead of following the regular visit schedule (which means that the patient might not meet with the adult provider for 6 months or more after transition), may ease the transition process and improve adherence.[171]

Personnel

Personnel are also required at each stage of the transition process from policy development to transition completion but are not used in the same way across transition programs. Some transition programs are separate, stand-alone clinics.[56,164-166] These programs require front-end, clinical, and back-end staff to support transition-related activities. Other transition programs exist within pediatric clinics and require personnel with transition-specific responsibilities such as a transition coordinator.[148,164,172-175] These programs must either hire staff whose responsibility is to manage transition processes or designate a portion of an existing staff member's responsibilities to transition-related tasks. Finally, other programs convene transition-related activities such as peer support or mentoring groups.[128,168] These programs also must hire staff to coordinate and provide services.

Given the diversity and complexity of young adults with special health care needs, a multidisciplinary approach to transition seems most likely to ensure a transition process that meets the range of medical, cognitive, and social needs.[51,57,61,87,111,138,144,151,176] Health care staff members involved in transition may include physicians, nurses, case managers, social workers, and peer mentors.[87,144,151] Nonetheless, the Society of Adolescent Medicine emphasizes the need for one designated professional to take responsibility for the process together with the patient and the family.[68] One of the more common suggestions is for that individual to be an assigned transition coordinator and advocate.[39,42,43,50,71,74,76,78,82,99,101,103,107,109,116,134,152,177]

A dedicated transition coordinator, either within the context of routine clinical care or in a specialized transition clinic, is a common approach to implementing a transition program.[66,75,78,79,82,98,101,108,109,122,134,148,164,169,171-175,178] This is also a role that is valued by patients and their families who consider the availability of a transition coordinator to be more important than paper-based resources.[134] The transition coordinator works with the transitioning youth to set developmentally appropriate goals, manage the transfer of information from the pediatric to adult provider, assist in making appointments with adult providers, arrange transportation, and facilitate the transfer from the family-centered orientation of pediatric care to the more individually oriented adult care system. The transition coordinator may attend the first adult appointment[78,122,169,171] and sometimes follows-up with the patient multiple times after transition to ensure that they are satisfied and receiving the care they need.[171] An advantage to assigning a care coordinator is that this staff member can assume a role that spans both pediatric and adult services as well as leverage already available community resources to meet individualized needs of transitioning youth.[69,98,122]

Several transition programs have reported using an advanced practice nurse as the transition coordinator,[69,108,117,120,141,144,151,164] with the theoretical advantages being their capacity to attain dedicated time for transition initiatives and their ability to serve as an expert, educator, researcher, leader, and consultant.[44,66,76,99,179] Alternatively, a community-based "navigator", or facilitator, offers the advantage of being unencumbered by an affiliation with any particular service system.[104,180]

Regardless of whether transition coordinators are used, both pediatric and adult providers and their staff need training in issues of adolescence.[36,89,151,181,182] Clinicians treating adolescents face specific challenges – particularly when the adolescent has special health care needs. These challenges may include determining the degree of autonomy versus family involvement appropriate to that individual, addressing risky behavior, and providing information in a way that is appropriate to their level of cognitive development (e.g., difficulties in considering long-term consequences of behaviors or nonadherence).

As is discussed in more detail in Guiding Question 2c, many providers (both adult and pediatric) do not receive specific training in providing care to adolescents and may be inadequately prepared to deal with adolescent issues such as puberty or lack of adherence to medication and treatment regimens because of the desire to be viewed the same as one's peers. For a transition program to be most effective, training in adolescent medicine can be helpful for the transition coordinator as well as for pediatric and adult primary care providers.

Further, pediatric providers may need training in transition processes and adult providers may need training in treatment of complex medical conditions beginning in childhood (e.g., cerebral palsy, Down syndrome, autism spectrum disorder); this is particularly true for adult physicians who treat patients with intellectual disabilities.[36,139] In cases where training the adult providers is not feasible, or the specific condition that a patient presents with is too rare to warrant training, the availability of consultation with experts in specific childhood-onset conditions may increase adult providers' willingness to provide care to transitioning youth with special health care needs.[124]

Perhaps the most important resource needed to implement high-quality transition care is a productive collaboration between pediatric and adult providers.[62,64,82,98,122,123,139,169-171] This collaboration can take different forms, such as scheduling one or a series of overlapping appointments with a pediatric and adult provider,[64,79,95,122] a joint clinic that includes both pediatric and adult providers,[61,98,109,170,180,183] or commencing appointments with an adult provider before transition.[57,120,134,169] Other effective strategies are having the pediatric provider attend the first appointment with the adult provider[170] and having the pediatric team followup with the transitioning youth after he or she has transitioned into adult care.[169,180]

Finally, trained personnel who are knowledgeable about the health insurance options available to transitioning youth with special health care needs are helpful to ensure that youth remain covered during the transition.[184] Adolescents and young adults with a chronic disease are less likely to have health insurance than any other age group,[169] and a trained staff person who can help them navigate changes in insurance coverage during the transition to adulthood can be valuable to avoid gaps in coverage or care. While the allowance for children to remain on parental insurance until age 26 and other expansions associated with the Affordable Care Act have the potential to mitigate some of these issues, it will still be important to provide support for navigating this changing benefits and access landscape.

Materials

Written guidelines[36,62,89,102,144,169,185,186] can include information such as the age at which transition should be initiated, the age by which certain behaviors are expected to have occurred, how youth readiness will be determined, as well as the specific staff responsibilities for different aspects of the transition process.[36,144]

Although written guidelines can serve as a type of transfer checklist, formal transfer checklists designed to guide pediatric provider actions and transfer knowledge to adult providers are also available.[50,62,79,82,171,187] A transfer checklist or plan might, for example, be kept on file with the pediatric provider and be sent to the adult provider. The plan may include information not necessarily contained in the medical record such as transition readiness, noncompliance issues, possible problems with insurance after transition, or other contextual factors.[78,171]

Information transfer ideally occurs well before the transition, so adult providers can understand the complications and challenges they might encounter.[62] Information transfer well in advance may be particularly important if the patient's condition is severe and requires emergency care after transitioning from pediatric care but before the first adult ambulatory visit. Transition checklists can also be useful in helping families prepare their son or daughter with special health care needs to take on more responsibility for his/her health care.[187]

Several tools have been proposed to assess patient readiness and may be incorporated into guidelines and checklists. These need to be acquired or developed at the clinic level. Examples include the Readiness to Transition Questionnaire[185] and a self-management scale to help providers determine how much of the youth's own care he or she has taken responsibility for (e.g., taking medications independently).[62] Another tool is The Transition Readiness Assessment Questionnaire (TRAQ), which incorporates the Transtheoretical Model for the five stages of change into a 5-point ordinal scale for measurement of completed transition tasks specifically for youth with special health care needs.[67] Disease specific transition readiness tools have also been developed for cystic fibrosis, cerebral palsy, and diabetes.[64,98,188] The Self-Management Scale, piloted to assess transition readiness in youth with cystic fibrosis, was found to be a better predictor than age for success in transfer to adult care.[62,64]

Additionally, for youth with special health care needs who also have an intellectual disability, an assessment of cognitive, developmental, and adaptive functioning will be critical in determining transition readiness, the optimal level of involvement by parents, and to inform adult providers.[51]

In addition to written guidelines, transfer checklists, and readiness assessments patient-and family-centered educational resources encouraging autonomy, self-advocacy, self-care responsibility, and treatment adherence may also be important.[50,78,87,89,144,187,189] Education materials that are available electronically, such as internet sites or mobile phone applications, are accessed more easily by young people.[92,126,135] Teens have also identified games, animation, messaging, and chat features as desirable features for such education materials.[135]

Workbooks used as learning tools can help providers assess the patients' knowledge and understanding of their disease process and transition needs.[83] Gilliam and colleagues[144] describe the development of a workbook for transitioning youth with HIV/AIDS that uses a developmental approach to teach and reinforce life skills and health information.

Education strategies are an important part of improving adherence and preparing the youth to be responsible for his or her care. Providers may tailor the specific approach to patient education based on the resources of the clinic and the needs of the population.

Tools for Transferring Knowledge Between Providers

Key Informants recommended that care plans be in place at the time of patient transfer. Similarly, the literature asserts that a system to transfer knowledge and information from the pediatric provider to the adult provider is important.[50,61,62,82,122,171,183,187,190,191] One example is the use of a transfer summary or checklist, kept on file with the pediatric provider and sent to the adult provider. The transfer summary or checklist includes important information not necessarily contained in the medical record such as a comprehensive summary of history of care, transition readiness, noncompliance issues, possible problems with insurance after transition, and recommendations for what might work best for the youth psychologically or physically.[61,122,171]

Towns and colleagues[62] noted that the transfer of information would ideally happen well before the transition actually occurs, so that the adult care team can have a full understanding of the extent of complications and challenges they might encounter. Having this transfer occur ahead of the first adult appointment could also be important if the youth with special health care needs requires emergency care after transitioning from pediatric care, but before their first ambulatory visit with the adult provider. Key Informants uniformly endorsed this idea.

Barriers to Implementation of Transition Care (Guiding Question 2c)

The literature describes several barriers to implementing transition care. We divided these barriers into systems and provider-related, and patient and family-related barriers.

Systems and Provider-Related Barriers

Cost and Insurance Problems

Changes in insurance and gaps in coverage are common in transition care, per the literature and the Key Informant interviews.[17,51,57,58,66,81,87,97,108,111,122,123,140,144,159,169,182,192-195] Key Informants noted that the challenges to implementing seamless transition of care are complicated by significant differences between pediatric and adult health care practice, stemming from issues related to coverage, eligibility, and other financial disincentives.

When children and adolescents age out of Medicaid eligibility or their parents' insurance, options for obtaining coverage may be limited or nonexistent,[108,140,193] and adolescents and young adults with special health care needs are less likely to have health insurance than any other age group.[169] Up to one-third of youth experience gaps greater than 6 months in health care coverage when moving from a pediatric to adult provider,[196] and between 15 and 30 percent of young adults with special health care needs have no insurance coverage.[14,193]

The age of transition often corresponds to a time when insurance coverage and benefits change. These insurance changes can result in decreased access to care for young adults and lack of coverage for those clinics that provide transition care further affecting reimbursement for services. Lack of insurance coverage during and after transition, as well as greater difficulties getting needed services for those receiving publically funded health care in adulthood [192] represents a significant barrier to implementing transition services, with serious implications for care throughout adulthood. Further, many young adults with special health care needs have difficulty maintaining employment, which can pose additional challenges to paying for health care. [122]

Health care providers are often held to benchmarked standards for volume of patients seen and levels of reimbursement within their practice. Transition care requires a significant amount of provider time, which results in a decrease in the number of patients seen by an individual provider.[78,111,189] However, this care does not result in a substantial increase in per visit reimbursement and can therefore translate into a financial loss to clinics that provide this type of service.[187]

In addition, transition care incorporates multidisciplinary services, which can be costly to those clinics that do not use these services for other patients. With the recent focus on pediatric medical homes, many pediatric clinics have greater access to multidisciplinary care,[123] so this cost difference might be more significant for the adult clinics typically designed for individual focused care.

Differences in the Culture of Pediatric Versus Adult Providers

Differences in how pediatric and adult clinics are structured, as well as in expectations for transitioning youth, may pose another barrier to effective transition care.[70,73,81,97,140,144,169,170,191,194,197] Given the initiation of the medical home concept in pediatric care, pediatric providers may be more accustomed to ensuring patients have followup appointments and prescription refills, whereas adult providers place more responsibility on the individual. Further, pediatric clinics may have greater familiarity with family-centered care, which is focused on developing a treatment plan that works for the youth with special health care needs and his or her family. Adult clinics, take a more patient-centered approach by treating the patient as an autonomous adult who makes his or her own informed decisions in collaboration with a provider[70,73,194] Although this emphasis on personal agency and self-sufficiency for adult patients compared with pediatric patients is developmentally appropriate, it can be difficult and overwhelming for the transitioning youth.[118,191] In particular, increasing emphasis on patient-centeredness in adult care, in which patients work in partnership with their clinicians to make health care decisions, may paradoxically cause undue stress on individuals with special health care needs especially as they transition.

The adult health care system currently tends to provide more fragmented care than the pediatric health care system, although an increasing emphasis on accountable care and models for implementing the adult medical home have significant potential to decrease fragmentation.[170] Medical and psychosocial services are particularly separate, and medical and psychiatric records are sometimes kept entirely distinct even within the same medical system, even though transitioning youth with special health care needs often have comorbid psychiatric disorders that need to be addressed in addition to their complex medical needs.[169] The need to make multiple appointments with different providers to get medical and psychosocial needs met through the adult care system, compared with the one-stop shop of pediatric providers, may pose a barrier to successful transition care. In particular, increasing emphasis on patient-centeredness in adult care, in which patients work in partnership with their clinicians to make health care decisions, may paradoxically cause undue stress on individuals with special health care needs especially as they transition.

Lack of Provider Training in Child-Onset Conditions

To some degree, adult providers lack in-depth training in childhood-onset conditions, having specialized in their training in adult medical care. Data from the literature support the Key Informant input that this is often the case; transitioning youth report that some adult providers do not have the skills or knowledge about childhood conditions to most effectively treat them.[29,87,100,108,162,191,192l,195,198,199]

This lack of knowledge can lead to reluctance by adult providers to accept responsibility for adolescents who have complex physical and psychological needs[70,113,124,144] leading to difficulty finding adult providers,[36,58,64,80,102,170,187,191] especially for youth with significant cognitive limitations.[51,170] As an example, in one study, more than half of pediatric neurologists were unable to find adult neurologists willing to care for patients with severe disabilities.[170]

Patient and Family-Related Barriers

Issues of Adolescent Development

Various developmental issues arise during adolescence that can be barriers to successful transition care.[64,65,79,81,87,97,100,106,159,169,182,194,200] Risky behavior, substance abuse, and concerns about sexual health all peak at this time. Furthermore, adolescence is a time when peers take on greater importance, and youth with special health care needs can make great effort to appear "normal" to their peers. Many adolescents have limited experience with financial independence or making their own decisions and may have difficulty keeping appointments and being responsible for their own health care. They may not have developed the skills to negotiate independently the adult service system, which is more complicated and fragmented than the pediatric system.[159] Many have not reached a level of maturity to be able to appreciate fully the long-term implications of their decisions.[64,200,201]

All of these behaviors, which are common to adolescence, can have a negative effect on the transitioning youth's ability to adhere to complicated medical regimens, and so are particularly troublesome for children with special health care needs.[14] Further, because most providers are trained to provide care to children or adults, few providers have training in how to treat adolescents, and it can be very difficult to know the most effective way to deliver care to this population.[134,144,151,159,194,202]

Finally, some youth with special health care needs have conditions that worsen in adolescence, such as increased difficulties with glycemic control for youth with diabetes[79,106] or the emergence of comorbid mental health problems, which are common among many youth with special health care needs.[57,106,194]

Problems With Adherence

Although likely confounded with issues of adolescent development (e.g., difficulty considering long-term implications of decisions and behaviors), differences in the structure of pediatric versus adult clinics (e.g., more hands-on followup to ensure adherence in pediatric clinics), or difficulties with insurance coverage, problems with adherence are common in transition-aged youth with special health care needs.[57,65,75,81,87,97,109,144,169,182,194,198,200] Problems can include forgetting to take medications, running out of medications, and not showing up for scheduled appointments. Some youth with special health care needs may feel "burnt out" on managing their conditions and might not seek maintenance care.[122]

Non-adherence is one of the leading causes of organ rejection, and older adolescents and young adults have the highest rates of non-adherence.[48,171,203] Young adult patients with diabetes have high rates of non-attendance after transfer to adult care and less frequent clinic contact is associated with poorer glucose control.[56,63,130] Youth with diabetes have higher rates of hospitalization because of acute hyperglycemia within two years after transfer.[23]

Resistance to Changing Providers

Youth and parents may resist changing providers.[51,66,70,75,81,82,87,97,100,118,122,169-171,182,191,195,197,199,204] It can be very difficult for families of youth with special health care needs to leave their familiar pediatric clinics for caregivers who are unfamiliar with their history,[66,70,87] and to "start over" and develop relationship with new providers.[51,73,108,204] Many youth express a preference for their pediatric providers and consider the adult service system to be impersonal.[100,122] Further, youth and their families express concern that the quality of care will not be as good in the adult setting as that they are receiving in the pediatric setting.[122,126,170,191,195,197] Reluctance about transitioning care to an adult provider can be compounded for youth who have medical conditions that carry with them stigma, such as HIV/AIDS.[57,144,169,182]

Resistance to changing health care providers can also occur on the part of the pediatric provider.[66,70,204] Pediatricians may be reluctant to transfer care to another physician who does not have a longstanding relationship with the youth with special health care needs, either because pediatricians feel that they can provide the best care for the youth and family, or because they are unaware of community and adult resources.

Other Barriers

Other barriers to implementing transition care are mentioned sporadically in the extant literature. Not properly assessing and understanding the implications of cognitive delays among youth with special health care needs can pose barriers to implementing successful transition care.[51,64,81,181] For these youth, providers must determine the extent to which parents should be involved in decisionmaking, and difficult behaviors (which are common among many youth with significant intellectual disability) may not be tolerated in adult provider offices.[170,183]

Similar issues arise for youth with physical disabilities, as parents may remain a critical part of decisionmaking if they provide substantial physical support.[205] Experiencing multiple other transitions at the same time as the health care transition, such as graduating from school, finding employment, moving out of the parental home, and starting a postsecondary education program, can be overwhelming to youth and affect their willingness to participate in transition programming.[73,195,198] Further, when youth with special health care needs attend a college program in another city, the physical distance between them and their primary care providers can be a barrier to successful transition care.[192,195] Finally, the lack of well-defined criteria for determining transition readiness makes decisions about when transition should begin difficult, especially if transition is initiated too early or too late.[73,109,194]

Delivery of Transition Interventions and Training (Guiding Question 2d)

Who Delivers Transition Interventions?

The National Heart, Lung and Blood Institute (NHLBI) recommends that transition teams include physicians, mid-level practitioners (e.g., nurses or physicians assistants), and social service workers from both pediatric and adult care settings.[87] Transition programs that take this multidisciplinary approach may have multiple team members who can address the array of complex needs experienced by youth with special health care needs.

Although the specific personnel in each of these programs differ, a common thread throughout is to assemble the personnel to address both the medical and psychological needs of youth with special health care needs as they transition, including experts in disease specific conditions, adolescent development, psychosocial considerations, and case management.[87,108]

Several examples of comprehensive transition programs have been described, each one tailored to meet the specific needs of the focus population or condition. A clinic for youth with chronic rheumatic disease, for example, includes a nurse specialist, physiotherapist, occupational therapist, social worker, and the availability of vocational and sexual health counseling in addition to the primary care providers.[64] A transition clinic for renal transplant patients includes a pediatric nephrologist, renal nurse, youth health specialist, renal pharmacist, renal dietician, and social worker.[89] A transition clinic for youth with sickle cell disease includes direct-care nurses, a nurse educator, clinical nurse specialist, nurse manager, physicians, social workers, case managers, pharmacists, and emergency staff.[151] Finally, one transition team for youth with HIV includes a case manager, social worker, health care provider, and youth advocate or peer partner.[144]

Depending on the specific needs of the youth, some of these professionals will play a more integral role in transition care, whereas others can be available for consultation as needed.[180,206] In some programs, an individualized team is assembled after assessing the needs of the transitioning youth.[141]

More common are transition programs whose personnel include one pediatric provider, one adult provider, and a mid-level provider who facilitates the transition between the pediatric and adult provider.[50,70,78,82,90,122,144,170] In these cases, the mid-level provider, often a nurse clinician, takes the role of the "transition specialist" by coordinating care from the pediatric to the adult provider and ensuring that the appropriate information is transferred. In one model, the nurse practitioner manages the care of the transitioning youth during his or her last years with the pediatric provider and then becomes the primary provider once the youth has transitioned to the adult care system.[144]

Although it is theoretically possible that the multidisciplinary team-based approach advocated by the NHLBI may result in better transition outcomes than programs that include health care providers only, these types of programs have not been tested against each other, and thus evidence for superiority is lacking. Resource barriers to implementation of team-based care in independent practices may be substantial, so practicality of this type of approach should also be studied.

What Additional Training is Necessary?

Ideally both pediatric and adult providers should receive training in issues of adolescence,[36,89,98,134,181,182,189] and at the least, the mid-level provider serving as the transition specialist should receive this training.[98,151] Further, for adult providers and for the transition specialist, additional training in complex conditions that begin in childhood (e.g., cerebral palsy, Down syndrome, autism spectrum disorder, congenital heart disease) is helpful;[29,141] this is particularly true for adult physicians who treat patients with intellectual disability.[36,139] Osterkamp and colleagues[181] describe an example of modules for training adult providers and include topics such as family-centered care, development of the healthy versus the chronically ill adolescent, and the Health Insurance Portability and Accountability Act. Training in adolescent medicine (to pediatric or adult providers) may address issues such as substance use, emotional wellbeing, and sexual health.[134] Callahan and colleagues[70] suggested that physicians trained in a medicine-pediatrics residency program might be particularly well suited to receive this type of training and to provide adult care to young adults with special health care needs.

Finally, because the transition specialist will need to work effectively with multiple providers and systems of care, training in how to promote collaboration among providers and team members may be helpful.[178]

27

Guiding Question 3. Description of the Existing Evidence (Evidence Map)

a. What patient groups/clinical conditions are represented in studies on the use and evaluation of transition care for children/adolescents with special health care needs?
b. What is the length of followup in studies on the use and evaluation of transition care for children/adolescents with special health care needs?
c. What outcomes are measured in studies on the use and evaluation of transition care for children/adolescents with special health care needs?

Patients and Conditions Represented in Evaluation Studies (Guiding Question 3a)

We identified 25[25,56,89,128,148-150,164-166,172-175,180,207-215, 239] studies reported in 30 publications[25,56,89,101,109,128,148-150,154,164-166,168,172-175,180,207-216, 239] that evaluated a system of purposeful transition care from the peer reviewed literature. We sought studies that measured effectiveness of a transition program and did not limit to any types of programs. This means we included studies of any approach to a system of transition care even if the evaluation outcome was defined as successful transfer, or if the system focused primarily on the transfer process. As discussed earlier in this technical brief, we use the term "transfer" generally to describe the point-in-time when a case is *transferred* from pediatric to adult care; we use the term "transition" to communicate a more comprehensive set of support processes and care that ideally begin before and extend some period of time after the moment of transfer. See Figure 1 for detailed reasons for exclusion.

Among the 25 studies, eight[56,150,164-166,173,210,213, 239] studied transition care for adolescents with diabetes. Five studies[25,89,172,174,207] studied transition care in adolescents who had undergone organ transplant; all but one of these focused on kidney transplant. Two studied transition care in sickle cell disease.[180,212] The remainder studied a variety of conditions including congenital adrenal hyperplasia,[149] HIV,[208] epilepsy,[209] juvenile idiopathic arthritis,[175] spina bifida,[214] cystic fibrosis,[148] inflammatory bowel disease,[215] or included a patient population comprising more than one chronic disease.[128, 211, 239]

Twelve studies were conducted in Europe: eight in the United Kingdom,[56,149,164,166,207,211,212,217] one in Germany,[25] one in Spain,[213] and two in Italy.[150,173] Eight studies were conducted in the United States;[128,148,165,174,180,212,214, 239] three studies were conducted in Canada;[89,168,209] and one study was conducted in Australia.[172] One study included data from the United Kingdom and Australia.[208] Interpretation of information from evaluation studies of transition care published in English from countries other than the United States must consider differences in the structure and financing of health care systems across countries.

Very few studies used a concurrent comparison group. Some studies compared survey responses of individuals who had participated in transition care with those of individuals who had not, with transition generally not occurring concurrently. This is because most interventions are implemented at the system level and provided to all relevant patients at the same time; thus, these studies generally relied on data from individuals who transitioned before the services were available as comparators.

Outcomes were generally patient-reported and focused mostly on issues such as satisfaction with the process or health-related quality of life. Some clinical outcomes are available in the literature; these include objective measures such as glycosylated hemoglobin (HbA1c) levels for patients with diabetes and rates of organ rejection among transplant patients. Generally, however, studies defined successful transition as attendance in adult care (transfer) or continued adherence to medication. Thus, although the programs offered comprehensive support rightly regarded as transition care, evaluations often focused on outcomes traditionally regarded as an index of the more limited concept of transfer.

In addition to the evaluation information on transition care for youth with special health needs that we found in the indexed literature, we catalogued relevant transition care resources, programs, and projects found in the gray literature. We include a detailed list of projects and resources in Appendix C and a summary of ongoing studies and funded projects in Appendix E.

Figure 1. Literature flow diagram

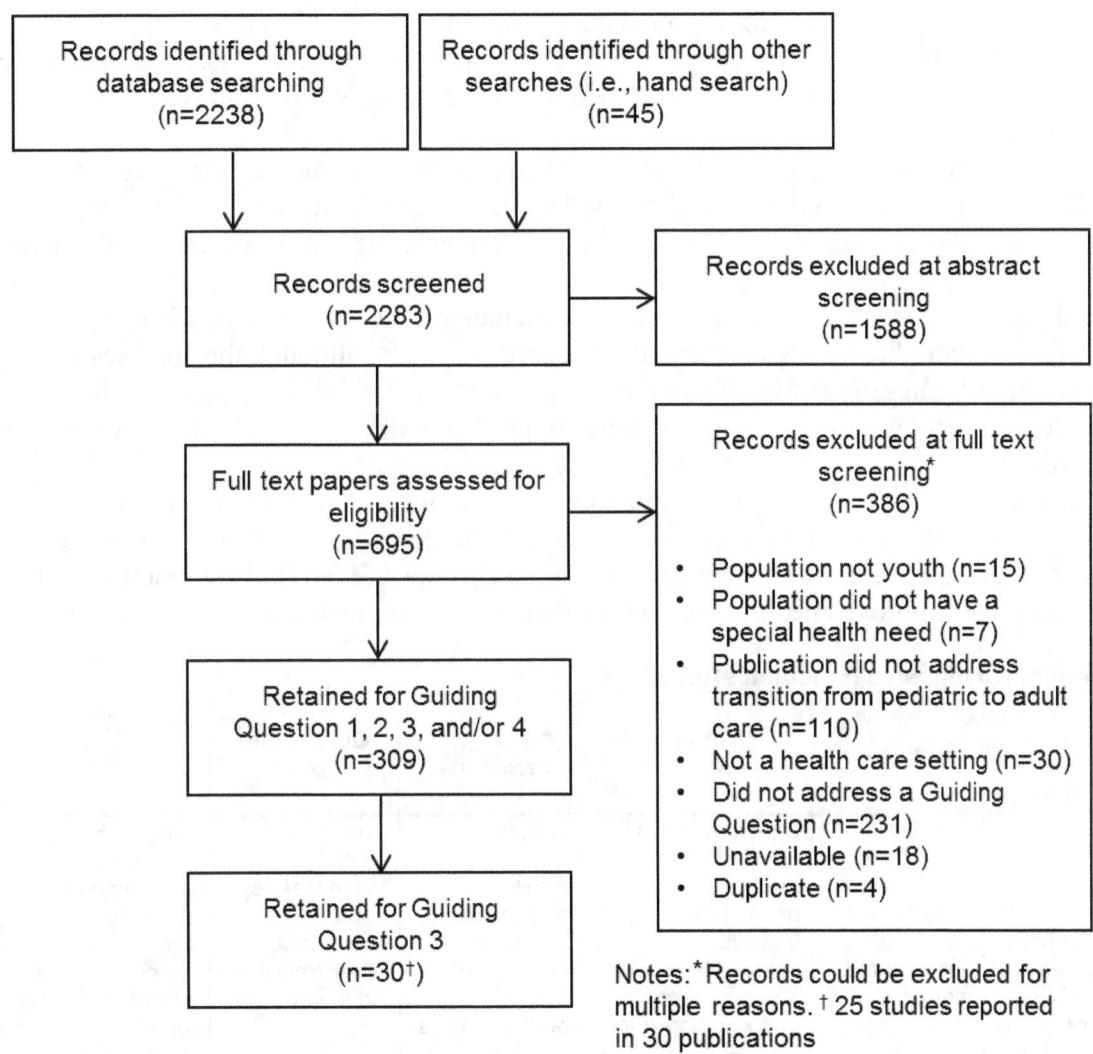

Notes: *Records could be excluded for multiple reasons. † 25 studies reported in 30 publications

29

Length of Followup (Guiding Question 3b) and Outcomes Measured (Guiding Question 3c) in Evaluation Studies

Diabetes

The most commonly studied group of transitioning youth was individuals with diabetes (Table 3). Numbers of young people with type I and type II diabetes have been steadily increasing,[218] and some evidence suggests that hormonal shifts in adolescence may complicate the maintenance of metabolic control.[219,220] Coupled with the need to participate in an adult health care system, maintaining good control in the transition to adulthood can be challenging in this population.

Transition care interventions studied to date have included use of a transition coordinator (n=2),[164,173] attendance of the pediatrician at the adult care visit(s) (n=2),[150,173] education and skill building (n=3),[165,166,213] a specialized young adult clinic (n=4),[56,164-166] and use of technology for education and reminders (n=2).[164,210] In five models, patients transferred directly into an adult clinic.[56,150,173,210,213] Practical assistance with scheduling was used in two programs.[164,213]

The most common diabetes-related outcomes were HbA1c levels (a marker for glycemic control),[56] diabetes-related hospitalizations,[164,210] and adult service attendance.[56,150,173,210] Seven studies used HbA1c levels as outcomes.[56,150,164-166,173,213] Patient satisfaction was the focus of two studies.[150,173]

None of the studies was entirely prospective. Five included some sort of comparison group,[56,165,166,173,210] with three using concurrent comparators,[56,165,173] although the analyses were retrospective. Three studies did not use a comparison group at all.[150,164,213] In general, studies were published as quality improvement evaluations, rather than with the intention of providing research inferences.

No two studies evaluated precisely the same transition care intervention, although some intervention components were common across studies. Nonetheless, there is clearly a need for replicated studies and for the use of concurrent comparison groups to identify best practices. All studies reported either improved health outcomes or maintenance of health.

Table 3. Overview of diabetes transition studies

Citation Location Study Description Length of Followup	Population	Transition Care Model	Setting(s)/ Provider(s)	Outcome(s) Reported	Results
Cadario F, et al., 2009[173] Italy Retrospective cohort (for identifying cases and collecting clinical data) with cross sectional survey data 1 year	Youth with type I diabetes in structured transfer plan (n=30) or unstructured method (n=32)	Structured transfer plan, including a designated pediatrician transition coordinator working with an endocrinologist to transfer care	Hospital Adult physicians, transition coordinator and endocrinologist	Date of first admission, mean HbA1c, clinic attendance rates, transition experience	Patients in the structured program had shorter transition, better clinic attendance and lower HbA1c. All reported favorable experience

Table 3. Overview of diabetes transition studies (continued)

Citation Location Study Description Length of Followup	Population	Transition Care Model	Setting(s)/ Provider(s)	Outcome(s) Reported	Results
Gholap N, et al., 2006[166] U.K. Retrospective comparison with data from another published study NR	Adolescents and young adults ages 16 to 25 with type I diabetes (n=68)	Young person's diabetes clinic that met monthly. Based on the Alphabet strategy, a mnemonic based approach to care: Advice; Blood Pressure lowering; Cholesterol and creatinine control; Diabetes control; Eye examination; Foot examination; use of Guardian drugs	Outpatient diabetes clinic (young person's diabetes clinic) Diabetologist, pediatrician, 2 "associate specialists", a pediatric and adult nurse specialist, a dietician and Asian link worker	Clinic attendance, HbA1c, hypertension, nephropathy, retinopathy, presence of complications	Patients who attended young person clinic had lower non-attendance (12% vs. 24.6%), lower mean HbA1c (8.4% vs. 9.5%), better blood pressure monitoring (100% vs. 88%), higher rates of screening for nephropathy, and lower rates of nephropathy (5% vs. 21%) compared with data from a recently published multicenter study.
Holmes-Walker DJ, et al., 2007[164] Australia Quality improvement assessment included retrospective collection of clinical data 12 months before participation and prospective data collection after clinic attendance. No comparison group. NR	Young adults with type I diabetes aged 15-25 years (n=191)	Transition coordinator or diabetes educator scheduled appointments for young people and provided reminders via phone, email or text; afterhours phone service was available	Young adult diabetes clinic within an adult referral hospital Diabetes educator Transition coordinator	Frequency of clinic visits, HbA1c, diabetic ketoacidosis, admissions	HbA1c improved significantly after a median of 5 visits (p<0.001); 82% attended clinics in the last 6 months; diabetic ketoacidosis admissions fell by 30%
Kipps S, et al., 2002[56] U.K. Retrospective cohort study of four regions, each of which employed a different transition approach Up to 2 years after transfer	Individuals with type I diabetes aged older than 18 years (n=229)	Four different transfer procedures at the district level: transfer from pediatric clinic to adult clinic, transfer to a young adult clinic, transfer with introduction to the adult provider before transfer, initial move to an adolescent clinic before moving to an adult clinic	4 health districts in the U.K. Young adult clinic	Age at transfer, clinic attendance rates, HbA1c	Clinic attendance dropped from 94% two years pre-transfer to 57% two years post transfer. Clinic attendance ranged from 29% to 71% across districts with higher rates among patients who met the adult provider before transfer

Table 3. Overview of diabetes transition studies (continued)

Citation Location Study Description Length of Followup	Population	Transition Care Model	Setting(s)/ Provider(s)	Outcome(s) Reported	Results
Lane JT, et al., 2007[165] Nebraska, U.S. Retrospective cohort study comparing outcomes in patients participating in the specialized clinic to patients who directly entered adult endocrine clinics 3 years	Young adults with type I diabetes aged 15 to 25 years seen in young adult clinic (n=96) or in general endocrine clinic (n=153)	Specialized clinic including an endocrinologist, 2 nurse educators and 2 dieticians. Services included substantial focus on education as well as group classes. The general endocrine clinic (comparison group) met in the same place and included a multidisciplinary provider team but without a class and with longer intervals between visits.	University diabetes center Specialized young adult diabetes clinic	Glycemic control measured via HbA1c	HbA1c levels did not change in either clinic overall. Within the highest tertile of HbA1c, patients in the young adult clinic had the largest decrease
Van Walleghem N, et al., 2006,[210] 2008,[168] and 2012[154] Manitoba, Canada Comparison of two cohorts – a younger group who had used the system, and an older group that had transferred before its implementation. Up to one year after referral to the program	Youth with type I diabetes aged under 18 years who participated in model (n=84) and older group aged 19-25 years who had transitioned without support (n=64)	Systems navigator model, administrative coordinator maintains phone and email contact with patients to identify barriers. Delivery methods include a comprehensive website, a bimonthly newsletter, a drop-in group, and educational events.	Community clinics, diabetes education resource center	Number of medical and diabetes educator visits, first year loss to follow up, diabetes-related hospitalizations, chronic complications, barriers to care in adult system	40% who did not have access to the navigator dropped out of medical care versus 11% who did
Vanelli M, et al., 2004[150] Cross sectional survey of patient experience, with pre-transition and post-transition HbA1c data collected from medical records. No comparison group. One year post transition and at study initiation	Adolescents with type I diabetes (n=73) with a mean age at transition of 21.0±0.95 years	Protocol for an uninterrupted procedure for transfer including introduction to the adult provider before transition and attendance by the pediatrician at the first adult visit. Transition occurred when the patient and parents agreed	Pediatric, adult specialty clinic Pediatric and adult providers	Patient satisfaction, attendance, HbA1c	94% of patients reported being satisfied with the process. Consensus about readiness to transition was achieved within 2 to 4 visits for 66% of patients. Mean HbA1c one-year post transition was 7.6±1,1% compared with 8.8±2.1% pre-transition

Table 3. Overview of diabetes transition studies (continued)

Citation Location Study Description Length of Followup	Population	Transition Care Model	Setting(s)/ Provider(s)	Outcome(s) Reported	Results
Vidal M, et al., 2004[213] Pre-post, no comparison group 1 year	Young adults with type I diabetes and a mean age of 19±1.3 years at transition (n=80)	Therapeutic Education Program for young adults transferring to adult care, including coordinated transfer visits, initial extended evaluation by adult staff (90 minutes), a pact to commit to the insulin therapy protocol with goal-setting, 4 group sessions with relatives, 3 to 6 individual visits over 6 months	Hospital-based adult outpatient clinic Adult endocrinologist and nurse; 12 to 15 hours dedicated to each patient, half of which were in group sessions	Meal plan composition, total daily insulin, HbA1c, body weight, number of hypoglycemic episodes	No changes in meal plan composition, no differences in daily insulin dose, increase in proportion of patients performing readjustments of insulin dose, decrease in HbA1c and in the number of hypoglycemic episodes

Abbreviations: HbA1c = Glycosylated hemoglobin; U.K. = United Kingdom; U.S. = United States

Solid Organ Transplant

A small body of literature[25,89,172,174,207] is available on the transition of pediatric patients with organ transplants to adult care (Table 4). Four of the five studies[25,89,172,207] focus on kidney transplant patients, with the remaining study[174] on liver transplant. All of the studies on kidney transplant patients include the evaluation of a specific transition oriented clinic – either one for youth alone or a joint pediatric-adult clinic. The one study on liver transplant patients evaluated the role of a transition coordinator.[174] This was the only prospective study, but the study did not use a concurrent control group, relying on historical comparators who had transitioned before implementation of the coordinator role.[174] The four studies on kidney transplant patients[25,89,172,207] report clinical outcomes, including organ rejection and mortality. The study on liver transplant patients[174] reports on patient satisfaction, psychological benefits, and medication adherence, confirmed via blood draw.

Table 4. Overview of transplant transition studies

Citation Location Study Description Length of Followup	Population	Transition Care Model	Setting(s)/ Provider(s)	Outcome(s) Reported	Results
Annunziato RA, et al., 2013[174] U.S. Prospective evaluation using historical (asynchronous) comparators who transferred before establishment of a transition coordinator 1 year	Patients in the pediatric liver transplant program (n=20) and historical cohort (n=14)	Transition coordinator who assisted with preparation, served as a liaison between pediatric and adult services, provided care coordination, provided outreach before and after transfer, and implemented research protocols to evaluate transition programming	Academic medical center; transition coordinator was a licensed clinical psychologist	Medication adherence measured via patient report and blood levels; Psychosocial outcomes including developmental skills and acceptability of the transfer process	Medication adherence was significantly better for patients who had access to the transition coordinator compared with the cohort who did not

Table 4. Overview of transplant transition studies (continued)

Citation Location Study Description Length of Followup	Population	Transition Care Model	Setting(s)/ Provider(s)	Outcome(s) Reported	Results
Chaturvedi S, et al., 2009[172] Australia Retrospective review of case notes followed by a patient survey 12 months	Pediatric kidney transplant recipients (n=11)	Transition clinic, development of self-management skills and a written transition summary	Children's hospital renal clinic Transition coordinator, transition adult nephrologist, and transition nurse	Serum creatinine levels, episodes of acute rejection, number of inpatient days, frequency of scheduled appointments and missed appointments	Patient health outcomes were fairly stable during the 12 months before and 12 months following transfer as measured by number of acute rejection episodes and hospital inpatient days. Adherence, as measured by attendance of scheduled appointments dropped from 73% before transfer to 57% after transfer

Table 4. Overview of transplant transition studies (continued)

Citation Location Study Description Length of Followup	Population	Transition Care Model	Setting(s)/ Provider(s)	Outcome(s) Reported	Results
Harden PN, et al., 2012,[207] and 2013[109] U.K. Comparison of two cohorts – a younger group who had used the system, and an older group that had transferred before its implementation Between 1 and 60 months after transfer	Young adult kidney transplant recipients (n=21); before 2006 (n=9); between 2006 and 2010 (n=12)	Integrated pediatric-young adult joint transition clinic and care pathway plus a young adult clinic located in a college sports center that included a youth worker. Patients are seen jointly by pediatric and adult teams from ages 15 – 18 and then transfer to the adult clinic at age 18. Patients are seen by providers without family members present to promote autonomy, and then meet with family members to review progress and management plans	Adult renal center and two pediatric renal centers (joint transition clinic)	Rates of acute organ rejection, morbidity, admissions	Six of nine patients who transitioned before implementation of the transition clinic had transplant failure compared with no transplant failures in the group that transferred after implementation of the transition clinic

36

Table 4. Overview of transplant transition studies (continued)

Citation Location Study Description Length of Followup	Population	Transition Care Model	Setting(s)/ Provider(s)	Outcome(s) Reported	Results
Pape L, et al., 2013[25] Germany Retrospective cohort One year prior and one year after transfer	Pediatric kidney transplant patients (n=66) in a transition clinic (n=15), patients transferred directly to an adult nephrologist (n=25), patients attending an adult nephrology clinic with a phase of alternate appointments over 1 to 2 years before transfer	Specialized transition clinic led by a specialized adult neurologist	Academic medical center (specialized transition clinic)	Survival, stability of immunosuppressive therapy, use of steroids and patient satisfaction	There was no difference in changes in clinical outcomes before and after transfer between the settings. Patient satisfaction was higher among those who transitioned via a specialized adolescent clinic compared with the patients who transferred to an adult nephrologist, either directly or by alternating appointments

Table 4. Overview of transplant transition studies (continued)

Citation Location Study Description Length of Followup	Population	Transition Care Model	Setting(s)/ Provider(s)	Outcome(s) Reported	Results
Prestidge et al., 2012[89] Canada System-level pre-post using historical controls 2 years	Kidney transplant recipients pre-transition clinic (n=34); transferred after opening transition clinic (n=12)	Multidisciplinary transition clinic where patients are seen every 4 to 6 months until transition in addition to attending standard transplant clinic. Transition team members see each patient. Specific educational goals include identifying the primary care provider, demonstrating medication knowledge, recognizing signs of rejection and infection, appraisal of ability to self-manage and awareness of reproductive health issues	Children's hospital, which is the referral center for renal transplantation in the region. Specialized transition clinic. Team includes a dedicated pediatric nephrologist, renal nurse, youth health specialist, renal pharmacist, renal dietician and social worker.	Deaths, allograft losses, graft function, costs per patient	The time to either graft loss or death was better for individuals transferred to adult care after implementation of the transition clinic than for individuals who transferred to adult care before implementation of the transition clinic. The average annual cost was less per patient for those who participated in the transition care clinic

Abbreviations: U.K. = United Kingdom; U.S. = United States

Other Conditions

We identified an additional 12 studies[128,148,149,175,180,208,209,211,212,214,215,239] on a range of conditions (Table 5). Two studies focused on sickle cell disease,[180,212] and three studies included patients with a variety of conditions,[128,211,239] while the remainder of the studies had one clinical focus.[148,149,175,208,209,214,215]

Two transition care interventions used a transition coordinator.[148,175] Five transition care interventions used multidisciplinary teams to provide care jointly,[148,180,208,211,215] and one evaluated a separate young adult clinic.[149] One transition care intervention provided direct scheduling of visits,[212] one was a mentoring group that met over 10 months,[128] and another used a generic 2 month intensive internet- and text message-based intervention followed by a 6 month review period.[239] Patient education was a common component of transition care.[128,148,175,180,209,214,215,239]

Table 5. Overview of other special health needs transition studies

Citation Location Study Description Length of Followup	Population	Transition Care Model	Setting(s)/ Provider(s)	Outcome(s) Reported	Results
Andemariam B, et al., 2013[180] Connecticut, U.S. Retrospective chart review After 5 years of implementation E+ only Outcome is transfer	Patients with sickle cell disease ages 16 to 24 years who began transition process between 2007-2012 (n=47)	Transition program combined between existing pediatric center with newly-formed adult center. Components included patient education, transitional phase included family meetings	Pediatric hospital and academic medical center	Demographics, clinical information (genotype, 3 year admission history for vaso-occlusive crisis or acute chest syndrome episodes, hydroxyurea or chronic transfusion therapy program), and transition clinic attendance.	68% patients had successfully transitioned. Risk factors for unsuccessful transition included: greater distance to travel and older age at time of initiation of transition. Patients with less severe disease (genotypes and no chronic transfusion therapy) were higher risk for unsuccessful transfer.
Bent N, et al., 2002[211] U.K. Cross sectional NA	Youth with longterm physical disability (n=245)	Young Adult Teams, including multidisciplinary teams including a consultant in rehabilitation medicine, a psychologist, therapists and a social worker	4 health care regions in the U.K., 2 with young adult team services and 2 with ad hoc services	Participation in society based on the international classification of functioning, disability and health	Individuals in the Young Adult Teams were more likely to participate in society than individuals who used ad hoc services

Table 5. Overview of other special health needs transition studies (continued)

Citation Location Study Description Length of Followup	Population	Transition Care Model	Setting(s)/ Provider(s)	Outcome(s) Reported	Results
Betz CL, et al., 2010[214] California, U.S. RCT 4 months followup	Youth with spina bifida, ages 14-18 years (n=65)	Transition Preparation Training, cognitive-behavioral program (8 sessions in a 2-day workshop) to facilitate development of transition plan	Academic children's hospital Training program administered by trainer	Well-being, role mastery, and self-care practice	No groups differences between groups
Bundock H, et al., 2011[208] U.K. and Australia Comparison of satisfaction with transition care among youth with HIV compared with youth with diabetes NR	Adolescents with perinatally acquired HIV in (n=21); Adolescents attending diabetes transition service (n=39)	Outpatient services using sequential approach to transition for HIV patients Outpatient clinic using direct transition model for patients with diabetes	Academic health science center clinic Pediatric infectious disease specialist, adult senior lecturer in HIV genitourinary medicine, adult HIV clinical nurse, adult psychologist	Patient satisfaction	Patients in both groups reported that transition from pediatric to adult care went smoothly and that transition was associated with improved health care
Chaudhry SR, et al., 2013[148] Michigan, U.S. Retrospective survey NA	Adults with cystic fibrosis (n=91) in a transition program vs. non-program participants	Structured transition program beginning early in adolescence, focusing on developing independence. Included a transition coordinator and participation of the adult pulmonologist in the pediatric clinic until readiness is achieved	Academic medical center	Patient satisfaction, perceived health status	Patient who went through a transition program were more satisfied with care before transferring to adult care
Gleeson H, et al., 2013[149] U.K. Retrospective record review NA	Individuals with congenital adrenal hyperplasia aged 16 years and older who attended pediatric clinic from 1992 to 2009 (n=61); pediatric clinics (n=37); Young Person Clinic (n=24)	Young Person Clinic at which the youth is introduced to an adult endocrinologist	Children's hospital Young Person Clinic had both pediatric and adult endocrine teams in attendance	Adult clinic attendance	Introduction of the Young Person Clinic had no effect on rates of engagement, with 50% lost to followup after transfer to adult services

Table 5. Overview of other special health needs transition studies (continued)

Citation Location Study Description Length of Followup	Population	Transition Care Model	Setting(s)/ Provider(s)	Outcome(s) Reported	Results
Greveson K, et al., 2011[215] London, U.K. Pre-post survey	Adolescents with inflammatory bowel disease (n=25)	Joint bimonthly transition clinic based on the Royal College of Nursing Model and including six key aspects: self-advocacy, sexual health, education and vocation, independent health care behavior, psychosocial support, and health and lifestyle. Adolescents enter at age 16 and remain in the transition service until the health care provider and parents agree that transfer to adult care is appropriate.	Pediatric specialty center	Time spent in transition clinic, patient knowledge of disease and factors important to transition	5 of the 21 pre-transfer respondents transferred to the adult service. Mean time spent in transition clinic was 8 months.
Hankins JS, et al., 2012[212] Tennessee, U.S. Pre-post pilot study 18 months preceding start of transition program and 18 months after start of the transition program	Youth with sickle cell disease aged 17 to 19 years (n=83)	Transition Pilot Program including a tour of adult SCD programs, lunch discussion with pediatric staff and scheduling of the first adult visit by the pediatric hematology case manager	Pediatric hospital Pediatric hematology staff	Proportion of pediatric patients fulfilling their first adult hematology appointment	Most (74%) of the transition program participants completed their first adult hematology appointment within 3 months as compared with 33% of those who did not participate in the transition program
Huang et al., 2014[239] California, U.S. Randomized Controlled Trial After the 8-month intervention	Youth ages 12-20 years with diabetes, inflammatory bowel disease, and cystic fibrosis (n=81)	Disease management intervention based on social cognitive theory and delivered via Web site and text messaging	Patient education (technology-based disease management) Pediatrician, public health educator	Disease self-management, health-related self-efficacy, patient-initiated communications, receipt of curriculum materials,	Relative to controls, transition program patients had improved disease management task performance, health-related self-efficacy, and patient-initiated communication

Table 5. Overview of other special health needs transition studies (continued)

Citation Location Study Description Length of Followup	Population	Transition Care Model	Setting(s)/ Provider(s)	Outcome(s) Reported	Results
Jurasek L, et al., 2010[209] Canada Cross sectional NA	Adolescents with epilepsy (n=97)	Nurse-led Adolescent Epilepsy Transition Clinic	Children's hospital	Patient satisfaction, understanding, and fears at 2 to 3 months after first visit	Patients and caregivers were satisfied with the transition process
Maslow G, et al., 2012[128] Rhode Island, U.S. Pre-post Length of time from pre- to post-test varied from 3 to 10 months One or more years following program participation (mean age of 20.6 years)	Individuals with a chronic illness (14 different conditions) aged 13 to 19 years (mean age 15.4 years) (n=20)	The Adolescent Leadership Council 10-month group mentoring program based on the Positive Youth Development framework	Children's hospital Pediatric and psychiatry residents, child life therapists, medical students, supervised by pediatric and psychiatry attending physicians; Had a fulltime director and clinical care was provided pro bono	Loneliness, chronic disease management, self-advocacy and successful transfer to adult care	Participants reported less loneliness and improved self-advocacy after participation in the mentoring program. There was a small increase in transition readiness scores for program participants
McDonough JE, et al., 2006a,[175] 2006b,[101] and Shaw KL, et al., 2006[216] U.K. Systems-level pre-post; Cross sectional 6 month followup 12 months after clinic visit	Adolescents with juvenile idiopathic arthritis aged 11 to 18 years (n=308)	Program of transitional care coordinated within each center with a program coordinator funded for one day per week. Patients worked through a series of templates that were developmentally appropriate and focused on home, health, and school. Informational resources were provided to patients and their families.	10 pediatric rheumatology centers	Satisfaction with care, health-related quality of life, and arthritis-related knowledge	Overall satisfaction scores improved significantly for adolescents and their parents after transition program implementation. Higher scores of acceptability for the local program coordinator compared with paper-based resources.

Abbreviations: NA = not applicable; NR = not reported; U.K. = United Kingdom

Guiding Question 4. Issues and Future Research

a. What are the implications (e.g., ethical, privacy, economic) of the current level of diffusion and of further diffusion of transition care for children/adolescents with special health care needs?

b. What are possible areas of future research for transition care for children/adolescents with special health care needs and which research designs are most appropriate to address these research topics?

Implications (Guiding Question 4a)

Documented decreases in adherence to medications and clinic appointments following transition are reasons to maximize successful transition.[23,203,221] Decreases in adherence are associated with worsening clinical outcomes including increased hospitalizations secondary to poorly controlled diabetes[23] and increased allograft loss in kidney transplant recipients[203] following transition, suggesting that the risks of unsuccessful transition are significant and that a paucity of transition programs could have substantial implications.

Poor reimbursement for transition services affects the ability of clinics to provide this care, which is often time intensive and multidisciplinary.[18,108,222] Up to 70 percent of physicians have reported that compensation adversely affected their ability to provide appropriate care for children with special health care needs because of lack of time, lack of patient insurance coverage and low reimbursement for the extra time required.[222] One review identified billing codes that can be used by clinicians to obtain appropriate reimbursement for these services, but it is unclear whether many or most physicians and coders are aware of how to use these codes appropriately.[223]

Given poor reimbursement and an overall dearth of transition programs, the reach and success of interventions may be affected by the income of the patient's family or type of insurance[14,18] as access to health care in the adult system is often limited for those patients with Medicaid insurance coverage.[170] Historically, the adolescent and young adult years marked a time during which a child was no longer covered under a parent's insurance.[224] This impact may be minimized in future years by the implementation of the Affordable Care Act in which individuals can remain on their parents' insurance plans up to age 26. Inequality exists in overall access to health care in the adult clinical setting with those of lower income or without private insurance receiving less access to health care, which affects medical care post-transition.[225]

Racial disparity may also occur, with some research suggesting that transition from pediatric to adult care is less successful in non-Hispanic black and Hispanic patients compared with Caucasian patients[14] and less successful in minority patients in general compared with Caucasians even in the setting of the pediatric medical home.[17,18] In addition, a higher familial education level has been associated with more successful transition, which may imply a lack of health literacy in the lower educated families whose educational needs are not met in the current transition systems.[18] Timing of transition may also affect medical outcomes after transition to adult care with one study of diabetic young adults suggesting that transfer to an adult clinic at a younger age was associated with worse outcomes.[133]

One barrier to successful transition is the lack of experience and training of adult clinicians in chronic diseases that were historically pediatric diseases.[45,54,68,191,226,227] In addition to the lack of experience of the clinicians, many adult clinics are not designed to treat adults with behavioral or developmental concerns, causing some to raise ethical concerns about whether it is appropriate to transition those patients to an adult provider unprepared to care for them.[170]

There are particular risks for patients with developmental or cognitive delay in that the current transition process most often involves an adult clinic, which has more of an individual focus rather than family focus when the patient's needs may require family-focused care.[45,170,228] Integrated systems of support for multidisciplinary care that are available in many pediatric

43

practices less often present in the adult clinic setting although the concept of the adult medical home is growing in concert with emphasis on population health and accountable care.[54,211,225,229]

Finally, developing transition programs will need to address the question of privacy as more providers and types of providers have access to the patient's medical information..[68,229,230]

In sum, the implications of the current diffusion of transition care are that many young people who need support in moving from pediatric to adult care are not receiving that support, and the adult system of care is unprepared to receive them. The risk of these patients falling through the cracks is substantial as they have serious and ongoing medical needs.

Areas for Future Research (Guiding Question 4b)

Methodologic and substantive issues should be addressed in future research about transition care. Methods issues include a common and validated definition of transition success, a need for more rigorous study designs, dedicated funding, and inclusion of a broader range of clinical research perspectives (i.e., involvement of pediatric and adult researchers). Areas and opportunities for future research include: technology, information about health care systems, disease progression, patient-specific transition, educational research, and cost research.

Definition of Successful Transition

A major barrier to transition research is a lack of well-defined outcome measures.[106,231-233] Possible metrics to evaluate success could include perceptions of success and satisfaction with the transition process (on the part of clinicians, adolescents, and parents), improved or stable disease-specific medical outcomes,[169,229] decreased or stable cost of health care, or educational milestones in a patient's ability to care for themselves or navigate the health care setting.[144,233,234] Without clear clinical or functional outcomes identified, most studies have focused on qualitative measures including clinicians' or patients' perceptions of success without objective measurements to support the claims of success of individual transition processes. No validated measures of transition have been developed.[231]

Future methodologic research should focus on identifying or developing objective measures of successful transition as well as transition tools.[114,161] Quality of life and personalized outcomes identified by the adolescents participating in transition care could be significant outcome measures, but others should be developed as well.[225,231-233,235] In addition, very few studies provided data on long-term followup, which could be important for considering the ultimate success of transitioning.

Study Design

Randomization in transition research can be problematic as medical care is multidisciplinary, and isolating any one intervention or holding constant concomitant interventions, even in a randomized controlled trial is difficult.[170,174,211,234] However, rigorous evaluation of these multidisciplinary transition programs is still needed.

Transition is a process often beginning in early adolescence and continuing through young adulthood. Ideally, researchers will design studies to evaluate participants before, during, and after the transition period. These studies would therefore need to be long, and thus may be cost prohibitive.[131,171,232,234] One method to obtain prospective data for evaluation of transition would be the development of disease-specific or location-specific core transition data sets that could be used for research of the transition process over the short term period as well as longitudinally.[234]

An alternative to using longitudinal studies to evaluate the impact of transition on patient outcomes and assess overall improvement in the transition process is quality improvement initiatives and evaluation designs.[20,59,236,237] Quality improvement research could help identify best practices for transition,[59] factors within transition that affect outcomes positively or negatively,[144,169,232] as well as individual predictors for successful transition.[169,232]

Funding

Funding streams generally focus on specific diseases, but the field of transition research would benefit from more generalized research that can identify effective methods across disease groups. Identifying funding streams that are nondisease specific may be challenging but important.[234]

Involvement of Pediatric and Adult Researchers

Traditionally, transition efforts and transition research has been led by pediatric providers even though adult providers are an essential component to the transition process. Future research should include both pediatric and adult researchers.[234] Research will also require involvement of primary care providers in addition to subspecialty care providers when applicable. No research has identified an optimal timing of transfer when multiple provider specialties are involved in an individual patient's care. Therefore, no data are available to guide which service should transfer first during the transition process.

Technology

The use of technology in transition has particular promise for adolescents, who tend to be comfortable users of technology. Novel uses of technology to improve adherence to medications, to provide education regarding their medical disease, to identify medical deterioration earlier, and to communicate with their health care providers should be further considered in future studies.[106,234,238-9] Given some of the disparities in access to care as children with special health care needs transition to adulthood may benefit from expansion and evaluation of uses of technology in the form of telemedicine.

One study reported improvement in medication adherence and decreased rejection in pediatric liver transplant patients who received text message reminders.[234] Another study also suggested that a disease generic intervention including text messaging components was associated with improvements in disease management task performance, health-related self-efficacy, and patient-provider communication,[239] but more research is needed in the area to confirm and expand on these concepts. In addition, the use of social media and its role in improving transition care would be an important area of research.

Information about Health Care Systems

A paucity of data exists regarding how individual systems affect transition. Transition programs would vary based on the health care system in which the care is provided. Some pediatric and adult clinic systems would share a core electronic medical record whereas other systems function more independently requiring development of standardized methods to communicate the complex medical history of the transitioning patients.

While research focusing on generalizable transition care processes is essential, the development of validated tools to aid a variety of systems in implementing successful transition is also necessary. Evaluations of transition care programs will need to specify the type of systems in which the transition was performed and what resources or tools were required to implement the program.

Documentation of resources could include specific programs such as city based transportation programs available to patients or clinic and institutional resources such as personnel, educational opportunities, and electronic medical record support. Identifying the differences and similarities within successful transition processes could be beneficial to the medical community as individual clinical systems modify components of the transition processes to work within their unique systems.

Natural Progression of Diseases

With improved clinical outcomes, many chronic diseases that were formerly seen only in pediatrics are now affecting adults. The adult course of these diseases is largely unknown, and therefore, aspects of transition specific for these diseases remain unclear. For these diseases, prospective tracking of the natural course and complications of these diseases will be necessary to determine what components of transition will be required when caring for adults with these diseases.[170,225,229]

Patient-Specific Information

Appropriate timing and necessary tools for successful transition may vary by severity or type of disease. Transition for individuals with a mildly debilitating disease could focus on disease self-management skills and medical system navigation whereas a transition program for individuals with severe disease may focus on palliative care and end of life challenges. The desired outcomes of the transition process could vary based on severity of disease as well.

Research of these programs would need to control for these differences in care and outcomes. In addition, the hypothesis that children with different diseases may require different transition processes requires further investigation since no study has evaluated the efficacy of disease specific versus general transition processes in a comparative manner.

Intellectual disability can be associated with some chronic diseases that affect children transitioning to adult care. The severity of disability influences the degree with which a young adult can manage their own care and therefore affects measures of successful transition. In addition, physical developmental delays or impairment can affect the ability of individuals to navigate the medical system independently. Successful research in transition would need to include stratification for cognitive ability and developmental delay for the subjects if variability exists. Future research efforts should evaluate the success of transition program modifications for patients with cognitive or physical impairments.

Behavioral health care is important in the transition process to provide support and services to address coping with chronic medical diseases and treatment, nonadherence, and psychological effects of their chronic disease. Few studies have addressed this aspect of transition care. Studies evaluating the role of behavioral health within the transition process will be critical.

Educational Research

As transition programs progress, one area of research that will be important is educational research to determine whether adult providers, multidisciplinary team members, adolescent providers, and developmental medicine providers are trained in the tenets of successful transition for adolescents with special health care needs.[44,93,131]

Educational research can also focus on the education provided to patients and parents throughout the transition process.[44,93,131,159]

Cost Research

We identified one cost study. The study took place in England so the relevance of the results to the United States health care system may be limited. The study did identify increased costs associated with the transition period, but did not find that an organized transition program was more resource intensive than ad hoc services.[211] Researchers should attempt to report the costs associated with transition implementation and service. This information can then be compared with the costs of unsuccessful transition in this patient population.[174,235]

Summary and Implications

The issue of how to provide good transition care for children with special health care needs warrants further attention. The numbers of children with special health care needs reaching adulthood are increasing, and the diversity of their clinical conditions is expanding. The Got Transition[38] resource provides a framework for transition care that can be adapted to serve the individual needs of a given patient population, but there is little evidence that it is used to provide a framework for evaluation in the research literature. Despite identifying numerous descriptions of existing transition programs or services, we identified only 24 evaluation studies.

Among the 25 studies, eight[56,150,164-166,168,173,210,213] studied transition care for adolescents with diabetes. Five studies[25,89,172,174,207] studied transition care in adolescents who had undergone organ transplant; all but one of these focused on kidney transplant. Two studied transition care in sickle cell disease.[180,212] The remainder studied a variety of conditions including congenital adrenal hyperplasia,[149] HIV,[208] epilepsy,[209] juvenile idiopathic arthritis,[175,216] spina bifida,[214] cystic fibrosis,[148] inflammatory bowel disease,[215] or included a patient population comprising more than one chronic disease.[128, 211, 239]

Twelve studies were conducted in Europe: eight in the United Kingdom,[56,149,164,166,207,211,212,217] one in Germany,[25] one in Spain,[213] and two in Italy.[150,173] Eight studies were conducted in the United States;[128,148,165,174,180,212,214,239] three studies were conducted in Canada;[89,168,209] and one study was conducted in Australia.[172] One study included data from the United Kingdom and Australia.[208] Interpretation of information from evaluation studies of transition care published in English from countries other than the United States must consider differences in the structure and financing of healthcare systems across countries.

Very few studies used a concurrent comparison group, although some compared survey responses of individuals who had participated in transition care with those of individuals who had not, with transition generally not occurring concurrently. This is because most interventions are implemented at the system level and provided to all relevant patients at the same time; thus, these studies generally relied on data from individuals who had previously transitioned before the services were available as comparators.

Outcomes were generally patient-reported and focused mostly on issues such as satisfaction with the process or health-related quality of life. Some clinical outcomes are available in the literature; these include objective measures such as glycosylated hemoglobin (HbA1c) levels for patients with diabetes and rates of organ rejection among transplant patients. Generally, however, successful transition is defined as attendance in adult care (transfer) or continued adherence to medication. Thus, although the programs offered comprehensive support rightly regarded as transition care, evaluation outcomes focused – at least in large part – on outcomes traditionally regarded as an index of the more limited concept of transfer.

Common components of care included use of a transition coordinator (6 studies), a special clinic for young adults in transition (8 studies) and provision of educational materials (12 studies), sometimes using computer-based programming.

Next Steps

Research needs are wide-ranging, including both substantive and methodologic concerns. At this point in time, the field lacks even a consistent and accepted way of measuring transition success, and it will be essential to establish consistent goals in order to build an adequate body of literature to affect practice.

One example of current efforts is The Health Care Transition Research Consortium, a volunteer organization of adolescent/young adult patients and health providers/researchers whose mission is to advance an evidence-based research agenda on health care transition. Stated goals include validated assessment tools to assess transition readiness, development and evaluation of interventions to improve transition process and disease self-management, and development of practice-based health care transition research networks (https://sites.google.com/site/healthcaretransition).

An important consideration going forward is recognizing that while the health care system as a whole should more uniformly address transition needs for children with special health care needs, the specific implementations will reflect the substantial heterogeneity of this population. For example, transition care for chronic conditions like diabetes may warrant a different approach than care provided for more heterogeneous and complex conditions, particularly those that include a behavioral or intellectual component. Care for some patients may be appropriately provided in primary care at the community level, while for others, it may be available only in highly specialized regional or academic centers. This heterogeneity and implications for approaches to transition care could form an important basis for research, including identifying predictors of successful transition as well as assessing the appropriateness of common elements of transition care for different conditions and identifying which elements should be different.

The impact of aging out of both Medicaid and Title V services for youth receiving them as children warrants consideration in development of transition plans, both in terms of educating youth and their families and in developing realistic plans for accessing care. As noted in the report, the concept of transition care in pediatrics is closely aligned with the medical home, and in fact, the "Got Transition" approach is built on the medical home concept. With implementation of the Affordable Care Act and increasing emphasis on coordinated care in accountable care organizations, there may be a natural place for transition services to be a part of new approaches to healthcare currently being piloted and implemented.

As noted in our brief, although Got Transition[38] principles are described by experts as the ideal basis for transition care, intervention studies are reported in such a way that we were unable to track back their interventions to these principles. If investigators would at minimum describe their interventions with the Got Transition[38] rubric—or another agreed upon rubric—then synthesizing the literature as it evolves would be more straightforward and enhance applicability.

Research on the costs and resources needed to provide good care will improve the likelihood of diffusion and may provide a basis for understanding reimbursement challenges. The broad availability of tools and materials to support providers and teams have the potential to reduce costs and increase provision of care.

References

1. A consensus statement on health care transitions for young adults with special health care needs. Pediatrics. 2002 Dec;110(6 Pt 2):1304-6. PMID: 12456949

2. McPherson M, Arango P, Fox H, et al. A new definition of children with special health care needs. Pediatrics. 1998 Jul;102(1 Pt 1):137-40. PMID: 9714637

3. Goodman DM, Hall M, Levin A, et al. Adults with chronic health conditions originating in childhood: inpatient experience in children's hospitals. Pediatrics. 2011 Jul;128(1):5-13. PMID: 21708805

4. Scal P, Ireland M. Addressing transition to adult health care for adolescents with special health care needs. Pediatrics. 2005 Jun;115(6):1607-12. PMID: 15930223

5. Neff JM, Anderson G. Protecting children with chronic illness in a competitive marketplace. JAMA. 1995 Dec 20;274(23):1866-9. PMID: 7500537

6. Newacheck PW, Kim SE. A national profile of health care utilization and expenditures for children with special health care needs. Arch Pediatr Adolesc Med. 2005 Jan;159(1):10-7. PMID: 15630052

7. Strickland BB, Singh GK, Kogan MD, et al. Access to the medical home: new findings from the 2005-2006 National Survey of Children with Special Health Care Needs. Pediatrics. 2009 Jun;123(6):e996-1004. PMID: 19482751

8. Transition of care provided for adolescents with special health care needs. American Academy of Pediatrics Committee on Children with Disabilities and Committee on Adolescence. Pediatrics. 1996 Dec;98(6 Pt 1):1203-6. PMID: 8951283

9. Gortmaker SL, Sappenfield W. Chronic childhood disorders: prevalence and impact. Pediatr Clin North Am. 1984 Feb;31(1):3-18. PMID: 6366717

10. Perrin JM, Bloom SR, Gortmaker SL. The increase of childhood chronic conditions in the United States. JAMA. 2007 Jun 27;297(24):2755-9. PMID: 17595277

11. Horner-Johnson W, Newton K. Using Population-Based Survey Data to Monitor the Health of Children and Youth with Special Health Care Needs and Disabilities. In: Hollar D, ed Handbook of Children with Special Health Care Needs. Springer New York; 2012:307-34.

12. Pollack L, McManus M. Special Analysis of the 2009/10 National Survey of Children with Special Health Care Needs by Lauren Pollack and Margaret McManus of the National Alliance to Advance Adolescent Health. March 2012

13. Stoeck PA, Cheng N, Berry AJ, et al. Health care transition counseling for youth with special health care needs. Am Fam Physician. 2012 Dec 1;86(11):1024. PMID: 23198669

14. McManus MA, Pollack LR, Cooley WC, et al. Current status of transition preparation among youth with special needs in the United States. Pediatrics. 2013 Jun;131(6):1090-7. PMID: 23669518

15. Toomey SL, Chien AT, Elliott MN, et al. Disparities in unmet need for care coordination: the national survey of children's health. Pediatrics. 2013 Feb;131(2):217-24. PMID: 23339228

16. Kane DJ, Kasehagen L, Punyko J, et al. What factors are associated with state performance on provision of transition services to CSHCN? Pediatrics. 2009 Dec;124 Suppl 4:S375-83. PMID: 19948602

17. Richmond N, Tran T, Berry S. Receipt of transition services within a medical home: do racial and geographic disparities exist? Matern Child Health J. 2011 Aug;15(6):742-52. PMID: 20602158

18. Richmond NE, Tran T, Berry S. Can the Medical Home eliminate racial and ethnic disparities for transition services among Youth with Special Health Care Needs? Matern Child Health J. 2012 May;16(4):824-33. PMID: 21505782

19. Reiss J. Health care transition for emerging adults with chronic health conditions and disabilities. Pediatr Ann. 2012 Oct;41(10):429-35. PMID: 23052147

20. White PH, McManus MA, McAllister JW, et al. A primary care quality improvement approach to health care transition. Pediatr Ann. 2012 May;41(5):e1-7. PMID: 22587507

21. Lotstein DS, McPherson M, Strickland B, et al. Transition planning for youth with special health care needs: results from the National Survey of Children with Special Health Care Needs. Pediatrics. 2005 Jun;115(6):1562-8. PMID: 15930217

22. Hazel E, Zhang X, Duffy CM, et al. High rates of unsuccessful transfer to adult care among young adults with juvenile idiopathic arthritis. Pediatr Rheumatol Online J. 2010;8:2. PMID: 20148143

23. Nakhla M, Daneman D, To T, et al. Transition to adult care for youths with diabetes mellitus: findings from a Universal Health Care System. Pediatrics. 2009 Dec;124(6):e1134-41. PMID: 19933731

24. Okumura MJ, Heisler M, Davis MM, et al. Comfort of general internists and general pediatricians in providing care for young adults with chronic illnesses of childhood. J Gen Intern Med. 2008 Oct;23(10):1621-7. PMID: 18661191

25. Pape L, Lammermuhle J, Oldhafer M, et al. Different models of transition to adult care after pediatric kidney transplantation: A comparative study. Pediatr Transplant. 2013 Sep;17(6):518-24. PMID: 23730905

26. Taylor A, Lizzi M, Marx A, et al. Implementing a care coordination program for children with special healthcare needs: partnering with families and providers. J Healthc Qual. 2013 Sep;35(5):70-7. PMID: 22913270

27. Schrander-Stumpel CT, Sinnema M, van den Hout L, et al. Healthcare transition in persons with intellectual disabilities: general issues, the Maastricht model, and Prader-Willi syndrome. Am J Med Genet C Semin Med Genet. 2007 Aug 15;145C(3):241-7. PMID: 17639594

28. Peter NG, Forke CM, Ginsburg KR, et al. Transition from pediatric to adult care: internists' perspectives. Pediatrics. 2009 Feb;123(2):417-23. PMID: 19171604

29. Patel MS, O'Hare K. Residency training in transition of youth with childhood-onset chronic disease. Pediatrics. 2010 Dec;126 Suppl 3:S190-3. PMID: 21123485

30. McManus M ea. Pediatric perspectives and Practices on Transitioning Adolescents with Special health Care Needs to Adult Health Care. Washington DC: National Alliance to Advance Adolescent Health. 2008

31. Callahan ST, Cooper WO. Continuity of health insurance coverage among young adults with disabilities. Pediatrics. 2007 Jun;119(6):1175-80. PMID: 17545386

32. National Center for Health Statistics. Healthy People 2010 Final Review: Disability and secondary conditions. U.S. Department of Health and Human Services. DHHS publication no. (PHS)2012–1038. Hyattsville, MD: 2012. : http://www.cdc.gov/nchs/healthy_people/hp2010/hp2010_final_review.htm

33. U.S. Department of Health and Human Services Health Resources and Services Administration Maternal and Child Health Bureau. The National Survey of Children with special health care needs chartbook 2005-2006. 2006

34. Bloom SR, Kuhlthau K, Van Cleave J, et al. Health care transition for youth with special health care needs. J Adolesc Health. 2012 Sep;51(3):213-9. PMID: 22921130

35. Patient Protection and Affordable Care Act. 42 USC § 18001 2010.

36. Cooley WC, Sagerman PJ. Supporting the health care transition from adolescence to adulthood in the medical home. Pediatrics. 2011 Jul;128(1):182-200. PMID: 21708806

37. Got Transition? Tools: Six Core Elements of Health Care Transition and Health Care Transition Index. http://www.gottransition.org/6-core-elements.

38. Got Transition? Center for Health Care Transition Improvement National Alliance to Advance Adolescent Health. http://www.gottransition.org/.

39. Rosen DS, Blum RW, Britto M, et al. Transition to adult health care for adolescents and young adults with chronic conditions: position paper of the Society for Adolescent Medicine. J Adolesc Health. 2003 Oct;33(4):309-11. PMID: 14519573

40. McDonagh JE, Foster HE, Hall MA, et al. Audit of rheumatology services for adolescents and young adults in the UK. British Paediatric Rheumatology Group. Rheumatology (Oxford). 2000 Jun;39(6):596-602. PMID: 10888703

41. Bobo N, Butler S. The transition from pediatric to adult diabetes health care. NASN Sch Nurse. 2010 May;25(3):114-5. PMID: 20486445

42. Bell LE, Sawyer SM. Transition of care to adult services for pediatric solid-organ transplant recipients. Pediatr Clin North Am. 2010 Apr;57(2):593-610, table of contents. PMID: 20371054

43. McDonagh JE. Growing up and moving on: transition from pediatric to adult care. Pediatr Transplant. 2005 Jun;9(3):364-72. PMID: 15910395

44. Shaw KL, Southwood TR, McDonagh JE. Transitional care for adolescents with juvenile idiopathic arthritis: a Delphi study. Rheumatology (Oxford). 2004 Aug;43(8):1000-6. PMID: 15150431

45. Scal P. Transition for youth with chronic conditions: primary care physicians' approaches. Pediatrics. 2002 Dec;110(6 Pt 2):1315-21. PMID: 12456951

46. Srivastava SA, Elkin SL, Bilton D. The transition of adolescents with chronic respiratory illness to adult care. Paediatr Respir Rev. 2012 Dec;13(4):230-5; quiz 5. PMID: 23069122

47. van Dyck PC, Kogan MD, McPherson MG, et al. Prevalence and characteristics of children with special health care needs. Arch Pediatr Adolesc Med. 2004 Sep;158(9):884-90. PMID: 15351754

48. Lerret SM, Menendez J, Weckwerth J, et al. Essential components of transition to adult transplant services: the transplant coordinators' perspective. Prog Transplant. 2012 Sep;22(3):252-8. PMID: 22951502

49. Schwartz LA, Tuchman LK, Hobbie WL, et al. A social-ecological model of readiness for transition to adult-oriented care for adolescents and young adults with chronic health conditions. Child Care Health Dev. 2011 Nov;37(6):883-95. PMID: 22007989

50. Grant C, Pan J. A comparison of five transition programmes for youth with chronic illness in Canada. Child Care Health Dev. 2011 Nov;37(6):815-20. PMID: 22007981

51. Herzer M, Goebel J, Cortina S. Transitioning cognitively impaired young patients with special health needs to adult-oriented care: collaboration between medical providers and pediatric psychologists. Curr Opin Pediatr. 2010 Oct;22(5):668-72. PMID: 20601881

52. Viner RM. Transition of care from paediatric to adult services: one part of improved health services for adolescents. Arch Dis Child. 2008 Feb;93(2):160-3. PMID: 17942588

53. Knauth A, Verstappen A, Reiss J, et al. Transition and transfer from pediatric to adult care of the young adult with complex congenital heart disease. Cardiol Clin. 2006 Nov;24(4):619-29, vi. PMID: 17098515

54. Pinzon JL, Jacobson K, Reiss J. Say goodbye and say hello: the transition from pediatric to adult gastroenterology. Can J Gastroenterol. 2004 Dec;18(12):735-42. PMID: 15605138

55. Betz CL. Nurse's role in promoting health transitions for adolescents and young adults with developmental disabilities. Nurs Clin North Am. 2003 Jun;38(2):271-89. PMID: 12914308

56. Kipps S, Bahu T, Ong K, et al. Current methods of transfer of young people with Type 1 diabetes to adult services. Diabet Med. 2002 Aug;19(8):649-54. PMID: 12147145

57. Cervia JS. Easing the Transition of HIV-Infected Adolescents to Adult Care. AIDS Patient Care STDS. 2013 Dec;27(12):692-6. PMID: 24073595

58. Ryan S. The adolescent and young adult with Klinefelter syndrome:ensuring successful transitions to adulthood. Pediatr Endocrinol Rev. 2010 Dec;8 Suppl 1:169-77. PMID: 21217609

59. Tuchman LK, Schwartz LA, Sawicki GS, et al. Cystic fibrosis and transition to adult medical care. Pediatrics. 2010 Mar;125(3):566-73. PMID: 20176665

60. Betz CL. Transition of adolescents with special health care needs: review and analysis of the literature. Issues Compr Pediatr Nurs. 2004 Jul-Sep;27(3):179-241. PMID: 15371115

61. Nobili RM, Duff AJ, Ullrich G, et al. Guiding principles on how to manage relevant psychological aspects within a CF team: interdisciplinary approaches. J Cyst Fibros. 2011 Jun;10 Suppl 2:S45-52. PMID: 21658641

62. Towns SJ, Bell SC. Transition of adolescents with cystic fibrosis from paediatric to adult care. Clin Respir J. 2011 Apr;5(2):64-75. PMID: 21410898

63. Kennedy A, Sloman F, Douglass JA, et al. Young people with chronic illness: the approach to transition. Intern Med J. 2007 Aug;37(8):555-60. PMID: 17640188

64. Robertson L. When should young people with chronic rheumatic disease move from paediatric to adult-centred care? Best Pract Res Clin Rheumatol. 2006 Apr;20(2):387-97. PMID: 16546063

65. Robb A, Findling RL. Challenges in the transition of care for adolescents with attention-deficit/hyperactivity disorder. Postgrad Med. 2013 Jul;125(4):131-40. PMID: 23933901

66. Jalkut MK, Allen PJ. Transition from pediatric to adult health care for adolescents with congenital heart disease: a review of the literature and clinical implications. Pediatr Nurs. 2009 Nov-Dec;35(6):381-7. PMID: 20166468

67. Sawicki GS, Lukens-Bull K, Yin X, et al. Measuring the transition readiness of youth with special healthcare needs: validation of the TRAQ--Transition Readiness Assessment Questionnaire. J Pediatr Psychol. 2011 Mar;36(2):160-71. PMID: 20040605

68. Suris JC, Akre C, Rutishauser C. How adult specialists deal with the principles of a successful transition. J Adolesc Health. 2009 Dec;45(6):551-5. PMID: 19931826

69. Betz CL, Redcay G. Creating Healthy Futures: an innovative nurse-managed transition clinic for adolescents and young adults with special health care needs. Pediatr Nurs. 2003 Jan-Feb;29(1):25-30. PMID: 12630502

70. Callahan ST, Winitzer RF, Keenan P. Transition from pediatric to adult-oriented health care: a challenge for patients with chronic disease. Curr Opin Pediatr. 2001 Aug;13(4):310-6. PMID: 11717554

71. Crowley R, Wolfe I, Lock K, et al. Improving the transition between paediatric and adult healthcare: a systematic review. Arch Dis Child. 2011 Jun;96(6):548-53. PMID: 21388969

72. Treadwell M, Telfair J, Gibson RW, et al. Transition from pediatric to adult care in sickle cell disease: establishing evidence-based practice and directions for research. Am J Hematol. 2011 Jan;86(1):116-20. PMID: 21061308

73. Fegran L, Hall EO, Uhrenfeldt L, et al. Adolescents' and young adults' transition experiences when transferring from paediatric to adult care: A qualitative metasynthesis. Int J Nurs Stud. 2014 Jan;51(1):123-35. PMID: 23490470

74. Hudsmith LE, Thorne SA. Transition of care from paediatric to adult services in cardiology. Arch Dis Child. 2007 Oct;92(10):927-30. PMID: 17895343

75. Eleftheriou D, Isenberg DA, Wedderburn LR, et al. The coming of age of adolescent rheumatology. Nat Rev Rheumatol. 2014 Jan 7PMID: 24394351

76. Kovacs AH, Verstappen A. The whole adult congenital heart disease patient. Prog Cardiovasc Dis. 2011 Jan-Feb;53(4):247-53. PMID: 21295666

77. Campbell T, Beer H, Wilkins R, et al. "I look forward. I feel insecure but I am ok with it". The experience of young HIV+ people attending transition preparation events: a qualitative investigation. AIDS Care. 2010 Feb;22(2):263-9. PMID: 20390505

78. Hilderson D, Westhovens R, Wouters C, et al. Rationale, design and baseline data of a mixed methods study examining the clinical impact of a brief transition programme for young people with juvenile idiopathic arthritis: the DON'T RETARD project. BMJ Open. 2013;3(12):e003591. PMID: 24302502

79. Lyons SK, Libman IM, Sperling MA. Diabetes in the adolescent: transitional issues. J Clin Endocrinol Metab. 2013 Dec;98(12):4639-45. PMID: 24152689

80. Swift KD, Sayal K, Hollis C. ADHD and transitions to adult mental health services: a scoping review. Child Care Health Dev. 2013 Oct 25PMID: 24164052

81. Lochridge J, Wolff J, Oliva M, et al. Perceptions of solid organ transplant recipients regarding self-care management and transitioning. Pediatr Nurs. 2013 Mar-Apr;39(2):81-9. PMID: 23705299

82. Kaufmann Rauen K, Sawin KJ, Bartelt T, et al. Transitioning adolescents and young adults with a chronic health condition to adult healthcare - an exemplar program. Rehabil Nurs. 2013 Mar-Apr;38(2):63-72. PMID: 23529944

83. Fair CD, Sullivan K, Gatto A. Best practices in transitioning youth with HIV: perspectives of pediatric and adult infectious disease care providers. Psychol Health Med. 2010 Oct;15(5):515-27. PMID: 20835962

84. Brumfield K, Lansbury G. Experiences of adolescents with cystic fibrosis during their transition from paediatric to adult health care: a qualitative study of young Australian adults. Disabil Rehabil. 2004 Feb 18;26(4):223-34. PMID: 15164956

85. Wiener LS, Kohrt BA, Battles HB, et al. The HIV experience: youth identified barriers for transitioning from pediatric to adult care. J Pediatr Psychol. 2011 Mar;36(2):141-54. PMID: 20040607

86. Majumdar S. The adolescent with sickle cell disease. Adolesc Med State Art Rev. 2013 Apr;24(1):295-306, xv. PMID: 23705531

87. Jordan L, Swerdlow P, Coates TD. Systematic review of transition from adolescent to adult care in patients with sickle cell disease. J Pediatr Hematol Oncol. 2013 Apr;35(3):165-9. PMID: 23511487

88. Sobota A, Neufeld EJ, Sprinz P, et al. Transition from pediatric to adult care for sickle cell disease: results of a survey of pediatric providers. Am J Hematol. 2011 Jun;86(6):512-5. PMID: 21594889

89. Prestidge C, Romann A, Djurdjev O, et al. Utility and cost of a renal transplant transition clinic. Pediatr Nephrol. 2012 Feb;27(2):295-302. PMID: 21823039

90. Webb N, Harden P, Lewis C, et al. Building consensus on transition of transplant patients from paediatric to adult healthcare. Arch Dis Child. 2010 Aug;95(8):606-11. PMID: 20515964

91. Bowen ME, Henske JA, Potter A. Health care transition in adolescents and young adults with diabetes. Clinical Diabetes. 2010;28(3):99-106.

92. Young S, Murphy CM, Coghill D. Avoiding the 'twilight zone': recommendations for the transition of services from adolescence to adulthood for young people with ADHD. BMC Psychiatry. 2011;11:174. PMID: 22051192

93. Mennito SH, Clark JK. Transition medicine: a review of current theory and practice. South Med J. 2010 Apr;103(4):339-42. PMID: 20224504

94. Tucker LB, Cabral DA. Transition of the adolescent patient with rheumatic disease: issues to consider. Pediatr Clin North Am. 2005 Apr;52(2):641-52, viii. PMID: 15820382

95. Betz CL. Health care transition for adolescents with special healthcare needs: where is nursing? Nurs Outlook. 2013 Sep-Oct;61(5):258-65. PMID: 23036691

96. Boyle MP, Farukhi Z, Nosky ML. Strategies for improving transition to adult cystic fibrosis care, based on patient and parent views. Pediatr Pulmonol. 2001 Dec;32(6):428-36. PMID: 11747245

97. Transitioning HIV-infected youth into adult health care. Pediatrics. 2013 Jul;132(1):192-7. PMID: 23796739

98. Gleeson H, Turner G. Transition to adult services. Arch Dis Child Educ Pract Ed. 2012 Jun;97(3):86-92. PMID: 21979963

99. Watson AR, Harden PN, Ferris ME, et al. Transition from pediatric to adult renal services: a consensus statement by the International Society of Nephrology (ISN) and the International Pediatric Nephrology Association (IPNA). Kidney Int. 2011 Oct;80(7):704-7. PMID: 21832978

100. Hanna KM, Woodward J. The transition from pediatric to adult diabetes care services. Clin Nurse Spec. 2013 May-Jun;27(3):132-45. PMID: 23575170

101. McDonagh JE, Shaw KL, Southwood TR. Growing up and moving on in rheumatology: development and preliminary evaluation of a transitional care programme for a multicentre cohort of adolescents with juvenile idiopathic arthritis. J Child Health Care. 2006 Mar;10(1):22-42. PMID: 16464931

102. Lebensburger JD, Bemrich-Stolz CJ, Howard TH. Barriers in transition from pediatrics to adult medicine in sickle cell anemia. J Blood Med. 2012;3:105-12. PMID: 23055784

103. McDonagh J, Gleeson H. Getting transition right for young people with diabetes. European Diabetes Nursing. 2011;8(1):24.

104. Stewart D. Transition to adult services for young people with disabilities: current evidence to guide future research. Dev Med Child Neurol. 2009 Oct;51 Suppl 4:169-73. PMID: 19740226

105. Tattersall RS. The MAGICC and practical approach to rheumatology transition. Br J Hosp Med (Lond). 2012 Oct;73(10):552-7. PMID: 23124284

106. Lewis K. All grown up: moving from pediatric to adult diabetes care. Am J Med Sci. 2013 Apr;345(4):278-83. PMID: 23531959

107. Ross HM, Fleck D. Clinical considerations for allied professionals: issues in transition to adult congenital heart disease programs. Heart Rhythm. 2007 Jun;4(6):811-3. PMID: 17556212

108. de Montalembert M, Guitton C. Transition from paediatric to adult care for patients with sickle cell disease. Br J Haematol. 2013 Dec 17PMID: 24345037

109. Harden PN, Sherston SN. Optimal management of young adult transplant recipients: the role of integrated multidisciplinary care and peer support. Ann Saudi Med. 2013 Sep-Oct;33(5):489-91. PMID: 24188944

110. Transition to adult care for youth with special health care needs. Paediatr Child Health. 2007 Nov;12(9):785-93. PMID: 19030468

111. Sobus KML, Karkos JB. Rehabilitation care and management for the individual with cerebral palsy, ages 13 through early adulthood. Critical Reviews in Physical & Rehabilitation Medicine. 2009;21(2):117-65.

112. Binks JA, Barden WS, Burke TA, et al. What do we really know about the transition to adult-centered health care? A focus on cerebral palsy and spina bifida. Arch Phys Med Rehabil. 2007 Aug;88(8):1064-73. PMID: 17678671

113. Reider-Demer M, Zielinski T, Carvajal S, et al. When is a pediatric patient no longer a pediatric patient? J Pediatr Health Care. 2008 Jul-Aug;22(4):267-9. PMID: 18590875

114. Viner R. Barriers and good practice in transition from paediatric to adult care. J R Soc Med. 2001;94 Suppl 40:2-4. PMID: 11601160

115. Greene S, Greene A. Changing from the paediatric to the adult service: guidance on the transition of care. Practical Diabetes International. 2005;22(2):41-5.

116. Sable C, Foster E, Uzark K, et al. Best practices in managing transition to adulthood for adolescents with congenital heart disease: the transition process and medical and psychosocial issues: a scientific statement from the American Heart Association. Circulation. 2011 Apr 5;123(13):1454-85. PMID: 21357825

117. Madge S, Bryon M. A model for transition from pediatric to adult care in cystic fibrosis. J Pediatr Nurs. 2002 Aug;17(4):283-8. PMID: 12219328

118. Betz CL, Lobo ML, Nehring WM, et al. Voices not heard: a systematic review of adolescents' and emerging adults' perspectives of health care transition. Nurs Outlook. 2013 Sep-Oct;61(5):311-36. PMID: 23876260

119. Berg Kelly K. Sustainable transition process for young people with chronic conditions: a narrative summary on achieved cooperation between paediatric and adult medical teams. Child Care Health Dev. 2011 Nov;37(6):800-5. PMID: 22007979

120. Parfitt G. Proving young person's experience transition: lessons from Wales. Paediatr Nurs. 2008 Nov;20(9):27-30. PMID: 19006948

121. Nazareth D, Walshaw M. Coming of age in cystic fibrosis - transition from paediatric to adult care. Clin Med. 2013 Oct;13(5):482-6. PMID: 24115706

122. Lewis-Gary MD. Transitioning to adult health care facilities for young adults with a chronic condition. Pediatr Nurs. 2001 Sep-Oct;27(5):521-4. PMID: 12025316

123. Lemly DC, Weitzman ER, O'Hare K. Advancing healthcare transitions in the medical home: tools for providers, families and adolescents with special healthcare needs. Curr Opin Pediatr. 2013 Aug;25(4):439-46. PMID: 23770924

124. Hall CL, Newell K, Taylor J, et al. 'Mind the gap'--mapping services for young people with ADHD transitioning from child to adult mental health services. BMC Psychiatry. 2013;13:186. PMID: 23842080

125. Shaw KL, Southwood TR, McDonagh JE. Developing a programme of transitional care for adolescents with juvenile idiopathic arthritis: results of a postal survey. Rheumatology (Oxford). 2004 Feb;43(2):211-9. PMID: 14523224

126. Applebaum MA, Lawson EF, von Scheven E. Perception of transition readiness and preferences for use of technology in transition programs: teens' ideas for the future. Int J Adolesc Med Health. 2013;25(2):119-25. PMID: 23740658

127. Christie D, Viner R. Chronic illness and transition: time for action. Adolesc Med State Art Rev. 2009 Dec;20(3):981-7, xi. PMID: 20653213

128. Maslow G, Adams C, Willis M, et al. An evaluation of a positive youth development program for adolescents with chronic illness. J Adolesc Health. 2013 Feb;52(2):179-85. PMID: 23332482

129. Amaria K, Stinson J, Cullen-Dean G, et al. Tools for addressing systems issues in transition. Healthc Q. 2011 Oct;14 Spec No 3:72-6. PMID: 22008577

130. Allen D, Cohen D, Hood K, et al. Continuity of care in the transition from child to adult diabetes services: a realistic evaluation study. J Health Serv Res Policy. 2012 Jul;17(3):140-8. PMID: 22767889

131. Ferris ME, Mahan JD. Pediatric chronic kidney disease and the process of health care transition. Semin Nephrol. 2009 Jul;29(4):435-44. PMID: 19615564

132. Duke NN, Scal PB. Adult care transitioning for adolescents with special health care needs: a pivotal role for family centered care. Matern Child Health J. 2011 Jan;15(1):98-105. PMID: 20012347

133. Helgeson VS, Reynolds KA, Snyder PR, et al. Characterizing the transition from paediatric to adult care among emerging adults with Type 1 diabetes. Diabet Med. 2013 May;30(5):610-5. PMID: 23157171

134. McDonagh JE, Shaw KL. Adolescent rheumatology transition care in the UK. Pediatr Ann. 2012 May;41(5):e8-15. PMID: 22587509

135. Breakey VR, Blanchette VS, Bolton-Maggs PH. Towards comprehensive care in transition for young people with haemophilia. Haemophilia. 2010 Nov;16(6):848-57. PMID: 20491954

136. Stille CJ. Communication, comanagement, and collaborative care for children and youth with special healthcare needs. Pediatr Ann. 2009 Sep;38(9):498-504. PMID: 19772236

137. Reiss J, Gibson R. Health care transition: destinations unknown. Pediatrics. 2002 Dec;110(6 Pt 2):1307-14. PMID: 12456950

138. Karas DJ, Costain G, Chow EW, et al. Perceived burden and neuropsychiatric morbidities in adults with 22q11.2 deletion syndrome. J Intellect Disabil Res. 2014 Feb;58(2):198-210. PMID: 23106770

139. Field B, Scheinberg A, Cruickshank A. Health care services for adults with cerebral palsy. Aust Fam Physician. 2010 Mar;39(3):165-7. PMID: 20369122

140. Monaghan M, Hilliard M, Sweenie R, et al. Transition readiness in adolescents and emerging adults with diabetes: the role of patient-provider communication. Curr Diab Rep. 2013 Dec;13(6):900-8. PMID: 24014075

141. Berg SK, Hertz PG. Outpatient nursing clinic for congenital heart disease patients: Copenhagen Transition Program. J Cardiovasc Nurs. 2007 Nov-Dec;22(6):488-92. PMID: 18090190

142. Stinson J, Kohut SA, Spiegel L, et al. A systematic review of transition readiness and transfer satisfaction measures for adolescents with chronic illness. Int J Adolesc Med Health. 2013 Jul 6:1-16. PMID: 23828488

143. Woodward JF, Swigonski NL, Ciccarelli MR. Assessing the health, functional characteristics, and health needs of youth attending a noncategorical transition support program. J Adolesc Health. 2012 Sep;51(3):272-8. PMID: 22921138

144. Gilliam PP, Ellen JM, Leonard L, et al. Transition of adolescents with HIV to adult care: characteristics and current practices of the adolescent trials network for HIV/AIDS interventions. J Assoc Nurses AIDS Care. 2011 Jul-Aug;22(4):283-94. PMID: 20541443

145. Paone MC, Wigle M, Saewyc E. The ON TRAC model for transitional care of adolescents. Prog Transplant. 2006 Dec;16(4):291-302. PMID: 17183935

146. Hait E, Arnold JH, Fishman LN. Educate, communicate, anticipate-practical recommendations for transitioning adolescents with IBD to adult health care. Inflamm Bowel Dis. 2006 Jan;12(1):70-3. PMID: 16374262

147. Wolfstadt J, Kaufman A, Levitin J, et al. The use and usefulness of My Health Passport: An online tool for the creation of a portable health summary. Int J Child Adolesc Health. 2010 2012-09-10;3(4):499-506.

148. Chaudhry SR, Keaton M, Nasr SZ. Evaluation of a cystic fibrosis transition program from pediatric to adult care. Pediatr Pulmonol. 2013 Jul;48(7):658-65. PMID: 22888094

149. Gleeson H, Davis J, Jones J, et al. The challenge of delivering endocrine care and successful transition to adult services in adolescents with congenital adrenal hyperplasia: experience in a single centre over 18 years. Clin Endocrinol (Oxf). 2013 Jan;78(1):23-8. PMID: 23009615

150. Vanelli M, Caronna S, Adinolfi B, et al. Effectiveness of an uninterrupted procedure to transfer adolescents with Type 1 diabetes from the Paediatric to the Adult Clinic held in the same hospital: eight-year experience with the Parma protocol. Diabetes Nutr Metab. 2004 Oct;17(5):304-8. PMID: 16295053

151. Cerns S, McCracken C, Rich C. Optimizing adolescent transition to adult care for sickle cell disease. Medsurg Nurs. 2013 Jul-Aug;22(4):255-7. PMID: 24147324

152. Rapley P, Davidson PM. Enough of the problem: a review of time for health care transition solutions for young adults with a chronic illness. J Clin Nurs. 2010 Feb;19(3-4):313-23. PMID: 20500270

153. Harris KM, Gordon-Larsen P, Chantala K, et al. Longitudinal trends in race/ethnic disparities in leading health indicators from adolescence to young adulthood. Arch Pediatr Adolesc Med. 2006 Jan;160(1):74-81. PMID: 16389215

154. Van Walleghem N, MacDonald CA, Dean HJ. Transition of care for young adults with type 1 and 2 diabetes. Pediatr Ann. 2012 May;41(5):e16-20. PMID: 22587508

155. Van Cleave J, Leslie LK. Approaching ADHD as a chronic condition: implications for long-term adherence. Pediatr Ann. 2008 Jan;37(1):19-26. PMID: 18240850

156. de Beaufort C, Jarosz-Chobot P, Frank M, et al. Transition from pediatric to adult diabetes care: smooth or slippery? Pediatr Diabetes. 2010 Feb;11(1):24-7. PMID: 20015124

157. Davis M, Geller JL, Hunt B. Within-state availability of transition-to-adulthood services for youths with serious mental health conditions. Psychiatr Serv. 2006 Nov;57(11):1594-9. PMID: 17085607

158. Burke R, Spoerri M, Price A, et al. Survey of primary care pediatricians on the transition and transfer of adolescents to adult health care. Clin Pediatr (Phila). 2008 May;47(4):347-54. PMID: 18180341

159. Park MJ, Adams SH, Irwin CE, Jr. Health care services and the transition to young adulthood: challenges and opportunities. Acad Pediatr. 2011 Mar-Apr;11(2):115-22. PMID: 21296043

160. Garvey KC, Wolpert HA, Rhodes ET, et al. Health care transition in patients with type 1 diabetes: young adult experiences and relationship to glycemic control. Diabetes Care. 2012 Aug;35(8):1716-22. PMID: 22699289

161. Wojciechowski EA, Hurtig A, Dorn L. A natural history study of adolescents and young adults with sickle cell disease as they transfer to adult care: a need for case management services. J Pediatr Nurs. 2002 Feb;17(1):18-27. PMID: 11891491

162. Oswald DP, Gilles DL, Cannady MS, et al. Youth with special health care needs: transition to adult health care services. Matern Child Health J. 2013 Dec;17(10):1744-52. PMID: 23160763

163. Parr JR, Jolleff N, Gray L, et al. Twenty years of research shows UK child development team provision still varies widely for children with disability. Child Care Health Dev. 2013 Nov;39(6):903-7. PMID: 23425219

164. Holmes-Walker DJ, Llewellyn AC, Farrell K. A transition care programme which improves diabetes control and reduces hospital admission rates in young adults with Type 1 diabetes aged 15-25 years. Diabet Med. 2007 Jul;24(7):764-9. PMID: 17535294

165. Lane JT, Ferguson A, Hall J, et al. Glycemic control over 3 years in a young adult clinic for patients with type 1 diabetes. Diabetes Res Clin Pract. 2007 Dec;78(3):385-91. PMID: 17602780

166. Gholap N, Pillai M, Virmani S, et al. The Alphabet Strategy and standards of care in young adults with type 1 diabetes. The British Journal of Diabetes & Vascular Disease. 2006 July 1, 2006;6(4):168-70.

167. Smith PE, Myson V, Gibbon F. A teenager epilepsy clinic: observational study. Eur J Neurol. 2002 Jul;9(4):373-6. PMID: 12099921

168. Van Walleghem N, Macdonald CA, Dean HJ. Evaluation of a systems navigator model for transition from pediatric to adult care for young adults with type 1 diabetes. Diabetes Care. 2008 Aug;31(8):1529-30. PMID: 18458141

169. Dowshen N, D'Angelo L. Health care transition for youth living with HIV/AIDS. Pediatrics. 2011 Oct;128(4):762-71. PMID: 21930548

170. Camfield PR, Gibson PA, Douglass LM. Strategies for transitioning to adult care for youth with Lennox-Gastaut syndrome and related disorders. Epilepsia. 2011 Aug;52 Suppl 5:21-7. PMID: 21790562

171. Annunziato RA, Hogan B, Barton C, et al. A translational and systemic approach to transferring liver transplant recipients from pediatric to adult-oriented care settings. Pediatr Transplant. 2010 Nov;14(7):823-9. PMID: 20609174

172. Chaturvedi S, Jones CL, Walker RG, et al. The transition of kidney transplant recipients: a work in progress. Pediatr Nephrol. 2009 May;24(5):1055-60. PMID: 19238453

173. Cadario F, Prodam F, Bellone S, et al. Transition process of patients with type 1 diabetes (T1DM) from paediatric to the adult health care service: a hospital-based approach. Clin Endocrinol (Oxf). 2009 Sep;71(3):346-50. PMID: 19178523

174. Annunziato RA, Baisley MC, Arrato N, et al. Strangers Headed to a Strange Land? A Pilot Study of Using a Transition Coordinator to Improve Transfer from Pediatric to Adult Services. J Pediatr. 2013 Aug 28PMID: 23993138

175. McDonagh JE, Southwood TR, Shaw KL. The impact of a coordinated transitional care programme on adolescents with juvenile idiopathic arthritis. Rheumatology (Oxford). 2007 Jan;46(1):161-8. PMID: 16790451

176. Groark CJ, McCall RB. Implementing Changes in Institutions to Improve Young Children's Development. Infant Ment Health J. 2011 Sep;32(5):509-25. PMID: 22114364

177. Musumadi L, Westerdale N, Appleby H. An overview of the effects of sickle cell disease in adolescents. Nursing Standard. 2012;26(26):35-40.

178. Rearick E. Enhancing success in transition service coordinators: use of transformational leadership. Prof Case Manag. 2007 Sep-Oct;12(5):283-7. PMID: 17885635

179. Higgins SS, Tong E. Transitioning adolescents with congenital heart disease into adult health care. Prog Cardiovasc Nurs. 2003 Spring;18(2):93-8. PMID: 12732802

180. Andemariam B, Owarish-Gross J, Grady J, et al. Identification of risk factors for an unsuccessful transition from pediatric to adult sickle cell disease care. Pediatr Blood Cancer. 2013 Dec 18PMID: 24347402

181. Osterkamp EM, Costanzo AJ, Ehrhardt BS, et al. Transition of care for adolescent patients with chronic illness: education for nurses. J Contin Educ Nurs. 2013 Jan;44(1):38-42. PMID: 23413447

182. Boudreau ME, Fisher CM. Providing effective medical and case management services to HIV-infected youth preparing to transition to adult care. J Assoc Nurses AIDS Care. 2012 Jul-Aug;23(4):318-28. PMID: 21820326

183. Camfield P, Camfield C, Pohlmann-Eden B. Transition from pediatric to adult epilepsy care: a difficult process marked by medical and social crisis. Epilepsy Curr. 2012 Jul;12(Suppl 3):13-21. PMID: 23476118

184. Nishikawa BR, Daaleman TP, Nageswaran S. Association of provider scope of practice with successful transition for youth with special health care needs. J Adolesc Health. 2011 Feb;48(2):209-11. PMID: 21257122

185. Gilleland J, Amaral S, Mee L, et al. Getting ready to leave: transition readiness in adolescent kidney transplant recipients. J Pediatr Psychol. 2012 Jan-Feb;37(1):85-96. PMID: 21878430

186. Meran S, Don K, Shah N, et al. Impact of chronic kidney disease management in primary care. QJM. 2011 Jan;104(1):27-34. PMID: 20805119

187. Jameson PL. Adolescent Transition: Challenges and Resources for the Diabetes Team. Diabetes Spectrum. 2011 2011 Winter;24(1):18-21.

188. Patton SR, Graham JL, Varlotta L, et al. Measuring self-care independence in children with cystic fibrosis: the Self-Care Independence Scale (SCIS). Pediatr Pulmonol. 2003 Aug;36(2):123-30. PMID: 12833491

189. McDonagh JE, Southwood TR, Shaw KL. Unmet education and training needs of rheumatology health professionals in adolescent health and transitional care. Rheumatology (Oxford). 2004 Jun;43(6):737-43. PMID: 14997008

190. Tong A, Jones J, Speerin R, et al. Consumer perspectives on pediatric rheumatology care and service delivery: a qualitative study. J Clin Rheumatol. 2013 Aug;19(5):234-40. PMID: 23872547

191. Lariviere-Bastien D, Bell E, Majnemer A, et al. Perspectives of young adults with cerebral palsy on transitioning from pediatric to adult healthcare systems. Semin Pediatr Neurol. 2013 Jun;20(2):154-9. PMID: 23948690

192. Montano CB, Young J. Discontinuity in the transition from pediatric to adult health care for patients with attention-deficit/hyperactivity disorder. Postgrad Med. 2012 Sep;124(5):23-32. PMID: 23095423

193. Goudie A, Carle AC. Ohio study shows that insurance coverage is critical for children with special health care needs as they transition to adulthood. Health Aff (Millwood). 2011 Dec;30(12):2382-90. PMID: 22147867

194.   Peters A, Laffel L. Diabetes care for emerging adults: recommendations for transition from pediatric to adult diabetes care systems: a position statement of the American Diabetes Association, with representation by the American College of Osteopathic Family Physicians, the American Academy of Pediatrics, the American Association of Clinical Endocrinologists, the American Osteopathic Association, the Centers for Disease Control and Prevention, Children with Diabetes, The Endocrine Society, the International Society for Pediatric and Adolescent Diabetes, Juvenile Diabetes Research Foundation International, the National Diabetes Education Program, and the Pediatric Endocrine Society (formerly Lawson Wilkins Pediatric Endocrine Society). Diabetes Care. 2011 Nov;34(11):2477-85. PMID: 22025785

195.   Packel L, Sood M, Gormley M, et al. A pilot study exploring the role of physical therapists and transition in care of pediatric patients with cystic fibrosis to the adult setting. Cardiopulm Phys Ther J. 2013 Mar;24(1):24-30. PMID: 23754936

196.   Garvey KC, Markowitz JT, Laffel LM. Transition to adult care for youth with type 1 diabetes. Curr Diab Rep. 2012 Oct;12(5):533-41. PMID: 22922877

197.   Coleman R, Moore S. Future considerations in the transition of paediatric neurodevelopmental patients to adult services. Australasian Journal of Neuroscience. 2006;18(1):15-20.

198.   Kreindler JL, Miller VA. Cystic fibrosis: addressing the transition from pediatric to adult-oriented health care. Patient Prefer Adherence. 2013;7:1221-6. PMID: 24376344

199.   Fernandes SM, Khairy P, Fishman L, et al. Referral patterns and perceived barriers to adult congenital heart disease care: results of a survey of U.S. pediatric cardiologists. J Am Coll Cardiol. 2012 Dec 11;60(23):2411-8. PMID: 23141490

200.   Bitsko MJ, Everhart RS, Rubin BK. The Adolescent with Asthma. Paediatr Respir Rev. 2013 Aug 21PMID: 23972334

201.   Van Lierde A, Menni F, Bedeschi MF, et al. Healthcare transition in patients with rare genetic disorders with and without developmental disability: neurofibromatosis 1 and Williams-Beuren syndrome. Am J Med Genet A. 2013 Jul;161a(7):1666-74. PMID: 23696535

202.   Vidqvist KL, Malin M, Varjolahti-Lehtinen T, et al. Disease activity of idiopathic juvenile arthritis continues through adolescence despite the use of biologic therapies. Rheumatology (Oxford). 2013 Nov;52(11):1999-2003. PMID: 23893666

203.   Shemesh E, Annunziato RA, Arnon R, et al. Adherence to medical recommendations and transition to adult services in pediatric transplant recipients. Curr Opin Organ Transplant. 2010 Jun;15(3):288-92. PMID: 20445451

204.   Woldorf JW. Transitioning adolescents with special healthcare needs: potential barriers and ethical conflicts. J Spec Pediatr Nurs. 2007 Jan;12(1):53-5. PMID: 17233668

205.   Stewart DA, Law MC, Rosenbaum P, et al. A qualitative study of the transition to adulthood for youth with physical disabilities. Phys Occup Ther Pediatr. 2001;21(4):3-21. PMID: 12043171

206.   Chamberlain MA, Kent RM. The needs of young people with disabilities in transition from paediatric to adult services. Eura Medicophys. 2005 Jun;41(2):111-23. PMID: 16200026

207.   Harden PN, Walsh G, Bandler N, et al. Bridging the gap: an integrated paediatric to adult clinical service for young adults with kidney failure. BMJ. 2012;344:e3718. PMID: 22661725

208.   Bundock H, Fidler S, Clarke S, et al. Crossing the divide: transition care services for young people with HIV-their views. AIDS Patient Care STDS. 2011 Aug;25(8):465-73. PMID: 21745141

209.   Jurasek L, Ray L, Quigley D. Development and implementation of an adolescent epilepsy transition clinic. J Neurosci Nurs. 2010 Aug;42(4):181-9. PMID: 20804112

210. Van Walleghem N, MacDonald CA, Dean HJ. Building connections for young adults with type 1 diabetes mellitus in Manitoba: feasibility and acceptability of a transition initiative. Chronic Dis Can. 2006;27(3):130-4. PMID: 17306065

211. Bent N, Tennant A, Swift T, et al. Team approach versus ad hoc health services for young people with physical disabilities: a retrospective cohort study. Lancet. 2002 Oct 26;360(9342):1280-6. PMID: 12414202

212. Hankins JS, Osarogiagbon R, Adams-Graves P, et al. A transition pilot program for adolescents with sickle cell disease. J Pediatr Health Care. 2012 Nov-Dec;26(6):e45-9. PMID: 22819193

213. Vidal M, Jansa M, Anguita C, et al. Impact of a special therapeutic education programme in patients transferred from a paediatric to an adult diabetes unit. European Diabetes Nursing. 2004;1(1):23-7.

214. Betz CL, Smith K, Macias K. Testing the transition preparation training program: A randomized controlled trial. Int J Child Adolesc Health. 2010;3(4):595-607. PMID: 22229060

215. Greveson K, Morgan N, Furman M, et al. Attitudes and experiences of adolescents in an innovative IBD transition service. Gastrointestinal Nursing. 2011;9(1):35-40.

216. Shaw KL, Southwood TR, McDonagh JE. Young people's satisfaction of transitional care in adolescent rheumatology in the UK. Child Care Health Dev. 2007 Jul;33(4):368-79. PMID: 17584391

217. Miller VA, Harris D. Measuring children's decision-making involvement regarding chronic illness management. J Pediatr Psychol. 2012 Apr;37(3):292-306. PMID: 22138318

218. Koike S, Takano Y, Iwashiro N, et al. A multimodal approach to investigate biomarkers for psychosis in a clinical setting: the integrative neuroimaging studies in schizophrenia targeting for early intervention and prevention (IN-STEP) project. Schizophr Res. 2013 Jan;143(1):116-24. PMID: 23219075

219. Amiel SA, Sherwin RS, Simonson DC, et al. Impaired insulin action in puberty. A contributing factor to poor glycemic control in adolescents with diabetes. N Engl J Med. 1986 Jul 24;315(4):215-9. PMID: 3523245

220. Urakami T, Suzuki J, Yoshida A, et al. Association between Sex, Age, Insulin Regimens and Glycemic Control in Children and Adolescents with Type 1 Diabetes. Clin Pediatr Endocrinol. 2010 Jan;19(1):1-6. PMID: 23926371

221. Lyons SK, Becker DJ, Helgeson VS. Transfer from pediatric to adult health care: effects on diabetes outcomes. Pediatr Diabetes. 2013 Dec 18PMID: 24350767

222. Davidson EJ, Silva TJ, Sofis LA, et al. The doctor's dilemma: challenges for the primary care physician caring for the child with special health care needs. Ambul Pediatr. 2002 May-Jun;2(3):218-23. PMID: 12014983

223. DeBaun MR, Telfair J. Transition and sickle cell disease. Pediatrics. 2012 Nov;130(5):926-35. PMID: 23027174

224. LaRosa C, Glah C, Baluarte HJ, et al. Solid-organ transplantation in childhood: transitioning to adult health care. Pediatrics. 2011 Apr;127(4):742-53. PMID: 21382946

225. Sawyer SM, Macnee S. Transition to adult health care for adolescents with spina bifida: research issues. Dev Disabil Res Rev. 2010;16(1):60-5. PMID: 20419772

226. Kaufman H, Horricks L, Kaufman M. Ethical considerations in transition. Int J Adolesc Med Health. 2010 Oct-Dec;22(4):453-9. PMID: 21404876

227. Kanter J, Kruse-Jarres R. Management of sickle cell disease from childhood through adulthood. Blood Rev. 2013 Nov;27(6):279-87. PMID: 24094945

228. Bailey S, O'Connell B, Pearce J. The transition from paediatric to adult health care services for young adults with a disability: an ethical perspective. Aust Health Rev. 2003;26(1):64-9. PMID: 15485375

229. Persson A, Newman C. When HIV-positive children grow up: a critical analysis of the transition literature in developed countries. Qual Health Res. 2012 May;22(5):656-67. PMID: 22218268

230. Van Deyk K, Moons P, Gewillig M, et al. Educational and behavioral issues in transitioning from pediatric cardiology to adult-centered health care. Nurs Clin North Am. 2004 Dec;39(4):755-68. PMID: 15561158

231. Watson R, Parr JR, Joyce C, et al. Models of transitional care for young people with complex health needs: a scoping review. Child Care Health Dev. 2011 Nov;37(6):780-91. PMID: 22007977

232. Fletcher-Johnston M, Marshall SK, Straatman L. Healthcare transitions for adolescents with chronic life-threatening conditions using a Delphi method to identify research priorities for clinicians and academics in Canada. Child Care Health Dev. 2011 Nov;37(6):875-82. PMID: 22007988

233. McLaughlin S, Bowering N, Crosby B, et al. Health care transition for adolescents with special health care needs: a report on the development and use of a clinical transition service. R I Med J (2013). 2013;96(4):25-7. PMID: 23641448

234. McDonagh JE, Kelly DA. The challenges and opportunities for transitional care research. Pediatr Transplant. 2010 Sep 1;14(6):688-700. PMID: 20557475

235. Beresford B. On the road to nowhere? Young disabled people and transition. Child Care Health Dev. 2004 Nov;30(6):581-7. PMID: 15527469

236. Grol R, Baker R, Moss F. Quality improvement research: understanding the science of change in health care. Qual Saf Health Care. 2002 Jun;11(2):110-1. PMID: 12448794

237. Grol R, Baker R, Moss F. Quality improvement research: understanding the science of change in healthcare. London: BMJ; 2004.

238. Weitzman ER, Kaci L, Quinn M, et al. Helping high-risk youth move through high-risk periods: personally controlled health records for improving social and health care transitions. J Diabetes Sci Technol. 2011 Jan;5(1):47-54. PMID: 21303624

239. Huang JS, Terrones L, Tompane T, et al. Preparing Adolescents With Chronic Disease for Transition to Adult Care: A Technology Program. Pediatrics. 2014 May 19. PMID: 24843066

Appendix A. Literature Search Strategies

Table A-1: Search strategy and results from PubMed (updated 9/5/2013)

	Search Terms	Search Results
#1	"Continuity of Patient Care"[mh:noexp] OR "Transition to Adult Care"[mh] OR transition[tiab] OR transitions[tiab] OR transitioning[tiab] OR transitional[tiab]	247658
#2	care[tiab] OR "healthcare"[tiab] OR "Health Services"[mh] OR "Health Services Research"[mh] OR "Health Services Accessibility"[mh] OR "Health Services Needs and Demand"[mh] OR "health services"[tiab] OR "Health Planning"[mh:noexp] OR "Patient Care Planning"[mh] OR "pediatric to adult"[tiab] OR "child to adult"[tiab]	2141964
#3	Adolescent[mh] OR youth[tiab] OR Child[mh] OR pediatric[tiab] OR paediatric[tiab] OR child[tiab] OR children[tiab] OR adolescent[tiab] OR adolescents[tiab] OR adolescence[tiab] OR teen[tiab] OR teens[tiab] OR teenage[tiab] OR teenager[tiab] OR teenagers[tiab] OR "Child Health Services"[mh] OR "Adolescent Health Services"[mh] OR "young people"[tiab]	2594321
#4	Adult[mh] OR adult[tiab] OR adults[tiab] OR adulthood[tiab]	5690952
#5	"Chronic Disease"[mh] OR "special needs"[tiab] OR "special healthcare needs"[tiab] OR "special health care needs"[tiab] OR "special health needs"[tiab] OR "Disabled Children"[mh] OR disability[tiab] OR disabled[tiab] OR "YSHCN"[tiab] OR "CSHCN"[tiab] OR "chronic disease"[tiab] OR "chronic illness"[tiab] OR "chronic diseases"[tiab] OR "Mental Disorders"[mh] OR "mental illness"[tiab] OR "attention deficit"[tiab] OR depression[tiab] OR anxiety[tiab] OR "conduct disorders"[tiab] OR autism[tiab] OR autistic[tiab] OR Asperger[tiab] OR Asperger's[tiab] OR "pervasive development disorders"[tiab] OR "Developmental Disabilities"[mh] OR "developmental delay"[tiab] OR "developmental delays"[tiab] OR "Intellectual Disability"[mh] OR "intellectual disabilities"[tiab] OR "mental retardation"[tiab] OR "mentally retarded"[tiab] OR asthma[mh] OR asthma*[tiab] OR diabetes[tiab] OR diabetic[tiab] OR "Diabetes Mellitus"[mh] OR Epilepsy[mh] OR "seizure disorders"[tiab] OR "seizure disorder"[tiab] OR epilepsy[tiab] OR "Headache Disorders"[mh] OR migraine*[tiab] OR "Brain Injuries"[mh] OR "traumatic brain injury"[tiab] OR "traumatic brain injuries"[tiab] OR concussion*[tiab] OR "Heart Defects, Congenital"[mh] OR "congenital heart disease"[tiab] OR "congenital heart defects"[tiab] OR "Hematologic Diseases"[mh] OR "blood disorders"[tiab] OR "sickle cell"[tiab] OR anemia[tiab] OR "HIV"[tiab] OR "HIV Infections"[mh] OR "Organ Transplantation"[mh] OR "transplant recipients"[tiab] OR "Deafness"[mh] OR "Blindness"[mh] OR deaf[tiab] OR blind[tiab] OR "Cystic Fibrosis"[mh] OR "cystic fibrosis"[tiab] OR "Cerebral Palsy"[mh] OR "cerebral palsy"[tiab] OR "Muscular Dystrophies"[mh] OR "muscular dystrophy"[tiab] OR "Down Syndrome"[mh] OR "Joint Diseases"[mh] OR arthritis[tiab] OR "functional disability"[tiab] OR "functional disabilities"[tiab] OR "Congenital, Hereditary, and Neonatal Diseases and Abnormalities"[mh] OR "congenital disease"[tiab] OR "congenital diseases"[tiab] OR "congenital defects"[tiab] OR "spina bifida"[tiab] OR "Crohn Disease"[tiab] OR Crohn[tiab] OR "Celiac Disease"[mh] OR celiac[tiab] OR "genetic disease"[tiab] OR "genetic disorder"[tiab] OR "genetic disorders"[tiab] OR "genetic diseases"[tiab]	4049292
#6	#1 AND #2 AND #3 AND #4 AND #5 NOT (comment[pt] OR letter[pt] OR editorial[pt] OR news[pt] OR patient education handout[pt] OR legal cases[pt] OR newspaper article[pt] OR news[pt] OR historical article[pt] OR jsubsetk)	1878
#7	#6 AND English[la] AND humans[mh]	1656
#8	#7 AND ("2000/01/01"[dp] : "3000/12/31"[dp])	1373

Key: [tiab] title or abstract word; [th] therapy; [la] language; [mh] medical subject heading; [pt] publication type; "jsubsetk" consumer health journal subset

Appendix B. Screening Forms

Table B-1. Abstract screening form

<table>
<tr><td colspan="4" align="center">**Abstract Screening Form**
Technical Brief Transition Care for Children with Special Health Needs</td></tr>
<tr><td colspan="4">First Author, Year: _____   Reference # _____</td></tr>
<tr><td colspan="4" align="center">**Primary Inclusion/Exclusion Criteria**</td></tr>
<tr><td>1. Population is children (youth)</td><td>Yes</td><td>No</td><td>Cannot Determine</td></tr>
<tr><td>2. Population with special health need (excluding end of life, palliative care, and cancer)</td><td>Yes</td><td>No</td><td>Cannot Determine</td></tr>
<tr><td>3. Addresses transition care from pediatric to adult</td><td>Yes</td><td>No</td><td>Cannot Determine</td></tr>
<tr><td>4. Health care setting</td><td>Yes</td><td>No</td><td>Cannot Determine</td></tr>
<tr><td>5. Reports original research</td><td>Yes</td><td>No</td><td>Cannot Determine</td></tr>
<tr><td>6. Addresses a guiding question</td><td>Yes</td><td>No</td><td>Cannot Determine</td></tr>
<tr><td colspan="4">
Retain for:
_____ **BACKGROUND/DISCUSSION** _____ **REVIEW OF REFERENCES** _____ **Other** _____

</td></tr>
<tr><td colspan="4">COMMENTS :

</td></tr>
</table>

Table B-2. Full text screening form

Full Text Screening Form
Transition Care for Children with Special Health Needs

First Author, Year: _____ Reference #_____

Inclusion/Exclusion Criteria		
1. Population is children (youth)	Yes	No
2. Population with special health need (exclude end of life, palliative care, cancer)	Yes	No
3. Addresses care transition from pediatric to adult	Yes	No
4. Healthcare setting	Yes	No
5. Reports original research	Yes	No

Addresses one or more of the following:

____GQ1a: What is the purpose of transition care and what are the theoretical advantages and disadvantages?
____GQ1b: What are the common components of transition care interventions or processes used in clinical practice for children/adolescents with special healthcare needs?
____GQ1c: How do currently used approaches to transitioning healthcare address the complexity of health issues including comorbidities and the presence of both physical and intellectual/developmental disabilities?
____GQ2a: How widely available are programs or approaches to transition care within the healthcare setting for children/adolescents with special healthcare needs?
____GQ2b: What are the resources needed to implement transition care?
____GQ2c: What are the specific barriers to implementing transition care or processes for children/adolescents with special healthcare needs?
____GQ2d: Who delivers transition interventions and what training is required to implement identified approaches to transition care for children/adolescents with special healthcare needs?
____*GQ3a: What patient groups/clinical conditions are represented in studies on the use and evaluation of transition care for children/adolescents with special healthcare needs?
____*GQ3b: What is the length of followup in studies on the use and evaluation of transition care for children/adolescents with special healthcare needs?
____*GQ3c: What outcomes are measured in studies on the use and evaluation of transition care for children/adolescents with special healthcare needs?
____GQ4a: What are the implications (e.g., ethical, privacy, economic) of the current level of diffusion and of further diffusion of transition care for children/adolescents with special healthcare needs?
____GQ4b: What are possible areas of future research for transition care for children/adolescents with special healthcare needs and what research designs are appropriate to address these research topics?
____Does not address a Guiding Question
*Must be original research evaluation study

Retain for:
_____ **REVIEW OF REFERENCES**   _____ **BACKGROUND/DISCUSSION**   _____Other

COMMENTS:

Appendix C. Summary of Gray Literature

Table C-1. Transition resources identified from Internet searches

Resource Name	Description	Organization/Institution	Condition	Consensus / Guideline	Portal	Patient Material	Clinician Guide	Fact Sheet / Data	Assessment / Evaluation Tool
Autism Transition Handbook: Health Care	Information on transition resources for individuals with autism spectrum disorder and links to state-level information.	Devereux Foundation	Autism		•	•			
Good2Go Transition Program	Program to prepare youth with chronic health conditions to leave the hospital by the age of 8 and use adult health care services successfully.	The Hospital for Sick Children	Chronic health condition		•	•			•
The Adolescent Leadership Council (TALC)	Mentor program for chronically ill adolescents to prepare for transition to adulthood.	Hasbro Children's Hospital	Chronic health condition		•	•			
Taking Responsibility for Adolescent/Adult Care (ON TRAC)	Model of transition care for adolescents with chronic health conditions.	Children's and Women's Health Centre	Congenital heart disease			•	•		•
Cystic Fibrosis Transition Program	Structured transition program.	University of Michigan	Cystic fibrosis			•			
Cystic Fibrosis Transition Program	Specialized service partners with patients family to facilitate transition to adult care.	Lurie Children's Memorial Hospital	Cystic fibrosis			•			
CART Model Programs	White paper discusses model programs for transition from childhood and adolescence to adult.	The Special Hope Foundation	Developmental disability			•	•		
Elizabeth M. Boggs Center on Developmental Disabilities	Developing a New Jersey Developmental Disabilities Transition to Adult Health Care Forum.	Rutgers Robert Wood Johnson Medical School	Developmental disability		•				

Resource Name	Description	Organization/Institution	Condition	Consensus / Guideline	Portal	Patient Material	Clinician Guide	Fact Sheet / Data	Assessment / Evaluation Tool
Florida Developmental Disabilities Council: Health Care Transition	Health care transition training modules, workbook, and other resources for young people with developmental disabilities.	Florida Developmental Disabilities Council	Developmental disability		•				
Moving from Pediatric to Adult Health Care, Healthy Transitions NY	Website developed for youth with developmental disabilities, family caregivers, service coordinators, and health care providers.	Golisano Children's Hospital, State University of New York Upstate Medical University	Developmental disability		•	•		•	
Special Hope Foundation	Foundation funds projects on delivery of health care to adults with developmental disabilities.	The Special Hope Foundation	Developmental disability		•				
Taking Charge of My Health: Partners in Transition	Special Hope Foundation funded project to develop and test training modules for parents of young adults with developmental disabilities through transition from pediatric to adult care.	Westchester Institute for Human Development	Developmental disability			•			
Tools for primary care providers	Provides a list of forms and tools to assist providers of adults with developmental disabilities.	Surrey Place Centre	Developmental disability						
The Maestro Project	A community resource and transition support service for young adults with type I and type II diabetes.	Department of Pediatrics and Child Health	Diabetes		•	•	•		
disability.gov	Federal government website catalogue of nationwide disability programs and services.	U.S. Department of Labor	Disability		•				
The Best Journey to Adult Life	Youth, family, and service providers identified best practices for transition to adulthood for youth with disabilities.	CanChild Centre for Childhood Disability Research, McMaster University	Disability	•		•	•		

Resource Name	Description	Organization/ Institution	Condition	Consensus / Guideline	Portal	Patient Material	Clinician Guide	Fact Sheet / Data	Assessment / Evaluation Tool
Transition Planning for Adolescents with Special Health Care Needs: Information for Families and Teens	Booklet for youth transitioning to adulthood with a section on health care issues.	Institute for Community Inclusion, University of Massachusetts	Disability		●	●		●	●
Transitioning Youth: Healthcare	Resources and tools to prepare youth with disabilities for health care transition.	Governor's Interagency Transition Council	Disability		●	●			
Work Ability Utah: Transition to Adult Health Care	Resources for assessment and planning of health care transitions for youth with special health care needs.	Utah Department of Health	Disability		●	●			●
Consensus statement on the management of GH-treated adolescent in the transition to adult care	Consensus workshop summary of transition for growth hormone treated patients in transition from pediatric to adult care.	European Society for Paediatric Endocrinology	Endocrine disease	●			●		
Young Person Clinic	Special clinic with pediatric and adult endocrine teams	Royal Manchester Children's Hospital	Endocrine disease			●			
Adolescent Epilepsy Transition Clinic	Nurse led transition clinic within an epilepsy program.	University of Alberta Hospital	Epilepsy			●	●		●
900 Clinic Transition Service	Specialty multidisciplinary clinic patients attend for 6-8 years.	Imperial College Healthcare NHS Trust	HIV			●			
Transition from CAMHS to adult mental health services (TRACK): a study of service organisation, policies, process and user and carer perspective	National Institutes for Health Research funded transition project on organizational and clinical determinants of effective transition from child and adolescent mental health services to adult psychiatric services.	University of Warwick	Mental health						●

Resource Name	Description	Organization/ Institution	Condition	Consensus / Guideline	Portal	Patient Material	Clinician Guide	Fact Sheet / Data	Assessment / Evaluation Tool
National Center for Medical Home Implementation: Transitions	Links to resources on appropriate care transitions, guidance documents, and opinion statements.	American Academy of Pediatrics	Not specified		•				
Transition to Adult Health Services	Information for providers and patients transitioning to adult health care.	Great Ormond Street Hospital for Children	Not specified			•	•	•	•
Improving Sickle Cell Transitions of Care through Health Information Technology	Ongoing project to understand the needs of Sickle cell disease patients, caregivers, and providers and create a toolkit for Sickle cell disease care transitions.	National Initiative for Children's Healthcare Quality (NICHQ)	Sickle cell disease		•				
Recommended Curriculum for Transition from Pediatric to Adult Medical Care for Adolescents with Sickle Cell Disease	Suggested topics, methods, and efficacy measurements and proposes steps for transitioning by age group with subsections on medical issues.	National Initiative for Children's Healthcare Quality (NICHQ)	Sickle cell disease	•			•		
Sickle Cell Disease Transition Program	Educational program coordinated by Child Life Specialist with didactic information, web-based and print resources.	Department of Pediatrics, Duke University	Sickle cell disease			•			•
Sickle Cell Disease Treatment Demonstration Program	Ongoing project of quality improvement strategies for care of individuals with sickle cell disease.	National Initiative for Children's Healthcare Quality (NICHQ)	Sickle cell disease		•				
Adolescent Health Transition Project	Information, links, and material on transition from pediatric to adult health care for adolescents with special health care needs.	Center on Human Development and Disability, University of Washington	Special health need		•	•	•	•	•

C-4

Resource Name	Description	Organization/Institution	Condition	Consensus / Guideline	Portal	Patient Material	Clinician Guide	Fact Sheet / Data	Assessment / Evaluation Tool
Adolescent Transition for People with Special Health Care Needs	Links to brochures summarizing transition, checklists for youth, and other resources.	Rhode Island Department of Health	Special health need			●	●	●	●
Catalyst Center: Youth Transition, Telemedicine and Other Capacity Building Services	Funded by Maternal and Child Health Bureau to support youth transition, telemedicine, and other capacity building services.	Catalyst Center, Boston University School of Public Health	Special health need		●				
Commission for Children with Special Health Care Needs: Transition Resources	Links to sites with information for helping young people with independence in health care	Kentucky Cabinet for Health and Family Services	Special health need		●				
Creating Healthy Futures (CHF clinic)	Transition clinic for adolescents and young adults with special health needs.	Department of Nursing, University of Southern California	Special health need				●		
Got Transition? Center for Health Care Transition Improvement	Guidance and tools to aid in health care transitions for adolescents and young adults.	The National Alliance to Advance Adolescent Health	Special health need	●	●	●	●	●	●
Health Transition Wisconsin	Web site with transition tools and links to additional resources for families and clinicians	Health Transition Wisconsin	Special health need		●	●	●		
Healthy and Ready to Work, National Resource Center	Includes resources for understanding systems, access to quality health care, and increasing involvement of youth.	Maternal and Child Health Bureau	Special health need		●	●			
Kentucky Youth Transitioning to Employment and Comprehensive Healthcare (KY TEACH)	Assist young people with special health care needs to find medical homes and employment with health insurance.	Kentucky Cabinet for Health and Family Services	Special health need		●	●			●

Resource Name	Description	Organization/ Institution	Condition	Consensus / Guideline	Portal	Patient Material	Clinician Guide	Fact Sheet / Data	Assessment / Evaluation Tool
Navigating Health Care Transitions	Information about pilot project and tool for recommendations by age group and life domain.	Family Voices Colorado	Special health need			●			
Office for Genetics & Children with Special Health Care Needs: Health Care Transition	Resource site for youth and providers, including an adult care notebook.	Maryland Department of Health and Mental Hygiene	Special health need		●	●	●		
Roadmap for Transitioning Adolescents from a Pediatric to an Adult Practice	Document developed by providers and parents to address transition from pediatric to adult care for patients with special health needs.	Children's Hospitals and Clinics of Minnesota	Special health need			●	●		
Special Medical Services: Health Care Transition	Description of planning process by the Specialized Medical Services and Health Care Transition Coalition to promote quality of care during the health care transition.	New Hampshire Department of Health and Human Services	Special health need	●		●	●	●	
Tools for Transition	Educational resources for youth, a transition resource directory, and health care transition checklist.	Massachusetts Family Voices	Special health need		●				
Transition Age Youth	Transition planning for adolescents with special health care needs and disabilities.	Massachusetts Child Psychiatry Access Project	Special health need			●	●		
Transition Information and Resources for Families and Youth	Transition resources for youth with special health care needs.	Louisiana Department of Health and Hospitals	Special health need		●				
Transition Program	Provides support for medically complex patients ready to transition from pediatric to adult care.	Lurie Children's Memorial Hospital	Special health need		●	●	●	●	

Resource Name	Description	Organization/ Institution	Condition	Consensus / Guideline	Portal	Patient Material	Clinician Guide	Fact Sheet / Data	Assessment / Evaluation Tool
Transition to Adult Health Care: A Training Guide in Two Parts	Workshop guide and materials for parents, and youth with special health care needs ready to transition to adult healthcare.	Waisman Center, University of Wisconsin Madison	Special health need			•		•	
Spina Bifida Transition Program	Describes processes, strategies, and tools to establish a transition program.	Children's Hospital of Wisconsin	Spina bifida				•		
				5	26	32	21	8	12

Data Coding and Definitions for Table C-1

Resource Characteristics

Resource Name: Name of resource
Description: Brief description
Organization / Institution: Name of organization, hospital, etc. and geographic location
Condition: Disease or condition of the target population

- cystic fibrosis
- congenital heart disease
- cerebral palsy
- diabetes
- any endocrine disease except diabetes (e.g. adrenal hyperplasia)
- HIV
- mental health
- any rheumatology disease (e.g., juvenile idiopathic arthritis)
- sickle cell disease
- special health need, may be generic or various
- transplant
- physical disability, may be generic or various
- developmental disability, may be generic or various
- chronic health condition except for those specified above, may be generic or various
- other
- not specified

Resource Components; coded as 0=no; 1=yes; X=unclear

Consensus / Guideline: Clear statements issued by organization or professional group usually identified as guideline, practice parameter, consensus statement, etc.
Portal: Links to various resources or materials
Patient Material: The resource or information targets the patient or the patient family
Clinician Guide: The resource of information targets the provider/ clinician
Facts / Data Sheet: May be specific or generic information on transition- may include statistics, facts, summary points- but is generally succinct.
Assessment / Evaluation Tool: Assessment or evaluation of transition readiness, transition process, or transition methods

Table C-2. U.S. Federal and State-level transition resources and programs

Title	Location	Description	Organization	URL
Achieving the Outcomes for CSHCN	HI	Transition to Adult Health Care, Work, & Independence is a major outcome of focus; section links to original guides and workbooks	State of Hawaii, Department of Health, Children with Special Health Needs Branch	http://health.hawaii.gov/cshcn/cshcnoutcomes/
Adolescent Services, Helping You Transition to Adulthood: Resources for New Jersey's Youth	NJ	Contains resource guides and outside resources for transitioning adolescents	New Jersey Department of Children and Families	http://www.nj.gov/dcf/adolescent/
Adolescent Transition for People with Special Health Care Needs	RI	Links to brochures summarizing transition, checklists for youth, Youth transition workbook (with section on healthcare advocacy), and other resources	State of Rhode Island Department of Health	http://www.health.ri.gov/specialhealthcareneeds/about/adolescenttransition/
Carolina Health and Transition (CHAT): A Guide to Transition from Pediatric to Adult Health Care	NC	Handbook for transitioning from pediatric to adult care	North Carolina Division of Public Health: Women's and Children's Health: Children and Youth	http://www.ncdhhs.gov/dph/wch/doc/lhd/CHAT/Youth_Guide_12-09.pdf
Commission for Children with Special Health Care Needs: Transition Resources	KY	Assist young people with special healthcare needs to find medical homes and employment with health insurance; create system changes that promote smooth transitions from school to work and from pediatric to adult healthcare; links to sites with information for helping young people with independence in health care.	Commission for Children with Special Health Care Needs, Kentucky Cabinet for Health and Family Services	http://chfs.ky.gov/ccshcn/ccshcntransition.htm
Continuum of Care	SC	Handbooks and manuals for transitioning to adulthood, with sections on health	Governor's Office of Executive Policy and Programs	http://www.oepp.sc.gov/coc/default.html
CSH Healthcare Transitioning	WY	Suggestions and resources for transitioning to adult health services	Wyoming Department of Health	http://www.health.wyo.gov/familyhealth/csh/transitions.html
DMH Transitional Age Youth Initiative	MA	Links to Young Adult Resource Guide with a section on health	Massachusetts Department of Mental Health	http://www.mass.gov/eohhs/gov/departments/dmh/transitional-age-youth-initiative.html
Health Care Program for Children with Special Needs (HCP)	CO	Page has a section that links to transition to adult health care resources - some created by state, some external	Colorado Department of Public Health and Environment	http://www.colorado.gov/cs/Satellite/CDPHE-PSD/CBON/1251617590646
Health Transition Wisconsin	WI	Web site with transition tools including videos, a checklist, and pocket guide, and links to additional resources for families and clinicians	Wisconsin Regional Centers, Children and Youth with Special Health Care Needs	http://www.healthtransitionwi.org/

Title	Location	Description	Organization	URL
Healthy and Ready to Work, National Resource Center	US	Website for a project that has ended, but includes resources for understanding systems, access to quality health care, and increasing involvement of youth.	Maternal and Child Health Bureau	http://www.syntiro.org/hrtw/
Independent Living Program	NV	Program with resources to prepare foster youth to transition to adulthood; medical care is one topic	Nevada Division of Child and Family Services	http://www.dcfs.state.nv.us/dcfs_independentliving.htm
Now that you're in high school... it's time to be more in charge of your health	FL	Booklet directs teens with SHN to be more in charge of their health care, focusing on both teens and the transition to adulthood	Florida Department of Health and University of FL	http://www.floridahealth.gov/alternatesites/cms-kids/kids_teens/documents/highschool_booklet.pdf
Office for Genetics & Children with Special Health Care Needs: Health Care Transition	MD	Office For Genetics And People With Special Health Care Needs resource site for youth and providers, including an adult care notebook	Maryland Department of Health and Mental Hygiene	http://phpa.dhmh.maryland.gov/genetics/SitePages/Health_Care_Transition.aspx
Oklahoma Healthy Transitions Initiative	OK	Initiative to establish consortium of statewide community-based services for transitioning youth; also has resource guides	Oklahoma Department of Mental Health and Substance Abuse Services	http://ok.gov/odmhsas/Mental_Health_/Children,_Youth,_and_Family_Services/Systems_of_Care/Oklahoma_Healthy_Transitions_Initiative_%28OHTI%29/
Special Education and Support Services: Secondary Transition	IL	Links to healthcare related webinar	Illinois State Board of Education	http://www.isbe.state.il.us/spec-ed/html/total.htm
Special Medical Services: Health Care Transition	NH	Description of planning process by the Specialized Medical Services and Health Care Transition Coalition to promote quality of care during the health care transition from adolescent to adult, including transition checklist and timeline for providers and other tools	New Hampshire Department of Health and Human Services	http://www.dhhs.state.nh.us/dcbcs/bds/sms/transition.htm
Systems in Sync: Transition to Adulthood	KS	Project focusing on guiding young adults with SHN through the transition to adulthood, specifically integrating health transition with work, education, and independent living.	Kansas Department of Health and Environment	http://www.systemsinsync.org/goals_transition.htm
Transition for Young Adults	DE	Page contains facts, principles, and local resources for transitioning	Healthy Delawareans with Disabilities	http://www.gohdwd.org/health-care/transition-for-young-adults/

Title	Location	Description	Organization	URL
Transition Guides	ID	Interactive guides to health care transition separated by age groups	Idaho Department of Health and Welfare	http://www.healthandwelfare.idaho.gov/Children/ChildrensSpecialHealthProgram/HealthCareTransitiontoAdulthood/tabid/1472/Default.aspx
Transition Health Care Checklist: Transition to Adult Living in Pennsylvania	PA	Checklist, resources, steps to assist youth and families in transitioning to adult health and health care	Pennsylvania Department of Health	http://www.portal.state.pa.us/portal/server.pt/community/special_kids_network/14205/transition_health_care_checklist/558090
Transition Information	TX	Information and links to resources for patients, patient families, and providers on transition of youth with special health needs from pediatric to adult care.	Texas Department of State Health Services	http://www.dshs.state.tx.us/cshcn/transinfo.shtm
Transition Information and Resources for Families and Youth	LA	Transition resources for youth with special health care needs, including a guide to family involvement and resources by state region	Louisiana Department of Health and Hospitals	http://dhh.louisiana.gov/index.cfm/page/1137
Transition Information Packet	IA	Booklet on transition for youth exiting the foster care system, with a section on health	Iowa Department of Human Services	http://www.dhs.iowa.gov/Consumers/Child_Welfare/Transition_Services/Transitioning%20to%20Adulthood.html
Transition Issues	OH	Links to a document on medical transition	Ohio Department of Health	http://www.odh.ohio.gov/odhprograms/cmh/cwmh/infofam/cmhfmtrn.aspx
Transition Resources	MT	Page of outside health care transition resources	Montana Department of Public Health and Human Services	http://www.dphhs.mt.gov/publichealth/cshs/transitionresources.shtml
Transition to Adulthood	MI	Page contains original guides and resource manuals for health care transition	Michigan Department of Community Health	http://www.michigan.gov/mdch/0,4612,7-132-2942_4911_35698-135030--,00.html
Transition to Adulthood	ND	Page has a section that links to external pediatric to adult health resources	North Dakota Department of Health, Children's Special Health Services	http://www.ndhealth.gov/cshs/TransitionToAdulthood.htm
Transitioning Youth: Healthcare	MD	Resources and tools to prepare youth with disabilities for health care transition	State of Maryland (collaboration of many departments)	http://www.mdtransition.org/Health%20Care.htm
Work Ability Utah: Transition to Adult Health Care	UT	Resources for assessing current status and planning health care transitions for youth with special health care needs	Utah Department of Health	http://www.workabilityutah.org/community/healthy/transitionhealthcare.php

Title	Location	Description	Organization	URL
Young Adults in Transition	OR	Links to a few resources for young adults in transition	Oregon Department of Human Services, Addiction and Mental Health Services	http://www.oregon.gov /oha/amh/pages/child-mh-soc-in-plan-grp/main.aspx#young
Young Adults Transition Plan: Your Future / Your Life	WA	Designed to guide youth towards adult life and additional responsibility in healthcare	Washington State Department of Health	http://here.doh.wa.gov/ materials/transition-plan-young-adults/13_CSHCN-18yr_E11L.pdf
Youth and Transition Services	MN	Resources for transitioning youth with mental health needs	Minnesota Department of Human Services	http://www.dhs.state.m n.us/main/idcplg?IdcS ervice=GET_DYNAMI C_CONVERSION&Re visionSelectionMethod =LatestReleased&dDo cName=dhs16_16720 9
Youth in Transition Grant	VT	Project to support youth transitioning to adulthood through community supports, events, resources - access to a medical home is one of the desired outcomes	Vermont Department of mental Health	http://www.youth-in-transition-grant.com/
Youth in Transition to Adulthood	TN	Links to a few resources and programs for transitioning youth, some for health and mental health	Tennessee Division of Mental Health Services	http://tn.gov/mental/chi ldren/child_youth_adul t.shtml
Youth Transitions, Office for Children with Special Health Care Needs	AZ	Page on government website that links to health transition resources	Arizona Department of Health Services	http://www.azdhs.gov/ phs/owch/ocshcn/yout h-transition.htm
Youth with Special Health Care Needs	CT	Page contains some original resources on transitioning to adult health care (for young adults, parents, and providers) and links to some external resources	Connecticut Department of Public Health	http://www.ct.gov/dph/ cwp/view.asp?a=3138 &q=432684

Table C-3. Consensus statements for transition care

Reference Organization(s) Country	Brief description
American Academy of Pediatrics, the American Academy of Family Physicians, and the American College of Physicians-American Society of Internal Medicine, 2002[1] A consensus statement on health care transitions for young adults with special health care needs United States	Critical first steps that the medical profession needs to take to realize the vision of a family-centered, continuous, comprehensive, coordinated, compassionate, and culturally competent health care system.
Bell et al., Adolescent transition to adult care in sold organ transplantation: a consensus conference report. (2008){#728} American Society of Transplantation, Pediatric Committee United States	Recommendations from a consensus conference for transition of children who have received solid organ transplants.
Clayton et al., Consensus statement on the management of the GH-treated adolescent in the transition to adult care. (2005){#1393} European Society of Paediatric Endocrinology, Consensus Development Conference England	Summary of discussions at a consensus workshop related to issues in caring for GH-treated patients in the transition from pediatric to adult life.
Nutt et al., Evidence-based guidelines for management of attention-deficit/hyperactivity disorder in adolescents in transition to adult services and in adults. (2007){#954} British Association for Psychopharmacology, Consensus Development Conference England	Consensus conference to review the body of evidence on childhood ADHD and the growing literature on ADHD in older age groups. Much of this initial guidance on managing ADHD in adolescents in transition and in adults is based on expert opinion derived from childhood evidence.
Peters and Laffel. Diabetes care for emerging adults: recommendations for transition from pediatric to adult diabetes care systems. (2011){#226} American Diabetes Association Transitions Working Group, Consensus Development Conference United States	Consensus statement provides a framework for health care delivery during the transition period and an agenda for future research for youth and young adults with diabetes and their health care providers.
Rosen et al., Transition to adult health care for adolescents and young adults with chronic conditions. (2003){#1194} Society for Adolescent Medicine United States	Endorsement of national consensus statement on Health Care Transitions for young adults with special health needs and additional recommendations from the Society for Adolescent Medicine.
Sable et al., Best practices in managing transition to adulthood for adolescents with congenital heart disease: the transition process and medical and psychosocial issues. (2011){#2204} American Heart Association United States	Recommendation for transition care for adolescents with congenital heart disease. Address timing, social and family dynamics, health supervision issues, and sexuality, pregnancy and reproductive issues.
Sullivan et al., Primary care of adults with developmental disabilities. (2011){#2205} Canadian Consensus Guidelines, Colloquium on Guidelines for the Primary Health Care of Adults with Developmental Disabilities (March 20, 2009) Canada	Colloquium on guidelines for the primary health care of adults with developmental disabilities held in March of 2009 updates the 2006 Canadian guidelines for primary care of adults with developmental disabilities.
Van Riper et al., Position of the American Dietetic Association: providing nutrition services for people with developmental disabilities and special health care needs. (2010){#1625} American Dietetic Association	Consensus statement developed by the panel of adult and pediatric nephrologists.

Reference Organization(s) Country	Brief description
United States	
Watson et al., Transition from pediatric to adult renal services. (2011){#1381} International Society of Nephrology; International Pediatric Nephrology Association, Consensus Development Conference United States	Consensus statement developed by the panel of adult and pediatric nephrologists.
Webb et al., Building consensus on transition of transplant patients from paediatric to adult healthcare. (2010){#480} Consensus Development Conference England	Seven consensus statements representative of the current opinion of families and the UK transplant community.

Table C-4. Description of selected transition programs

Citation Location	Model	Population	Setting	Description
Jurasek et al., 2010[7] Edmonton, Canada **	**Adolescent Epilepsy Transition Clinic**	Epilepsy	University of Alberta Hospital	Nurse-led transition clinic within comprehensive epilepsy program
Kripke et al., 2011[8] California, U.S.	**CART model program**	Developmental disability	Administered by public health insurance plan	Includes medical home, center of excellence, and health advocacy services
Betz and Redcay, 2003[9] California, U.S.	**Creating Healthy Futures**	Special health care needs	Department of Nursing Clinic, University of Southern California	Family nurse practitioner, interagency team of child and adult providers
Amaria et al., 2011[10] Toronto, ON, Canada	**Good2Go Transition Program**	Chronic health conditions	The Hospital for Sick Children	Preparation for youth with chronic health conditions to leave the hospital and use adult healthcare services successfully
Paone, et al., 2006[11] British Columbia	**ON TRAC**	Pediatric transplant	Children's and Women's Health Care Centre	Developmentally appropriate (based upon adolescent development) teaching including tasks and skills and a care pathway to outline management practice and quality transitional care.
Kaufmann Rauen et al., 2013[12] Wisconsin, U.S.	**Spina Bifida Transition Program**	Spina bifida	Children's hospital	Partnership between pediatric and adult providers, guided by the Transition Care Model and the Ecological Model of Secondary Conditions and Adaptation
Stewart, et al. 2009[13] Hamilton, ON, Canada	**The Best Journey to Adult Life**	Developmental disability	CanChild Centre for Childhood Disability Research, McMaster University	Best practices for the transition to adulthood for youth with disabilities

Citation Location	Model	Population	Setting	Description
Smith et al., 2011[14] North Carolina, U.S.	**Sickle Cell Disease Transition**	Sickle cell disease	Duke Department of Pediatrics	Coordinated by a child life specialist
Vanelli et al., 2004[15] **	**Parma protocol**	Adolescents with type 1 diabetes	Pediatric, adult specialty clinic Pediatric and adult providers	Protocol for an uninterrupted procedure for transfer including introduction to the adult provider prior to transition and attendance by the pediatrician at the first adult visit. Transition occurred when the patient and parents agreed
Chaudhry et al., 2013[16] Michigan, U.S. **	**Structured transition program**	Adults with cystic fibrosis	Academic medical center	Structured transition program beginning early in adolescence, focusing on developing independence. Included a transition coordinator and participation of the adult pulmonologist in the pediatric clinic until readiness is achieved.
Gerber et al., 2007[17] Illinois, US	**STYLE**	Young adults with diabetes	Inner-city clinics and childhood diabetes registry Diabetes educator	Internet-based transition program including information on DM, goal-setting exercises with feedback, role-playing, empowerment and communication skills
Maslow et al., 2012[18] Rhode Island, U.S. **	**The Adolescent Leadership Council (TALC)**	Individuals with a chronic illness aged 13-19 years	Hasbro Children's hospital Pediatric and psychiatry residents, child life therapists, medical students, supervised by pediatric and psychiatry attending physicians	10-month group mentoring program based on the Positive Youth Development framework
Van Walleghem et al., 2006[19] and 2008[20] Manitoba, Canada **	**The Maestro Project**	Youth with type 1 diabetes aged under 18 years	Community clinics, diabetes education resource center	Systems navigator model, administrative coordinator maintains phone and email contact with patients to identify barriers. Delivery methods include a comprehensive website, a bimonthly newsletter, a drop-in group and educational events
Hankins et al., 2012[21] Tennessee, U.S. **	**Transition Pilot Program**	Youth with sickle cell disease aged 17-19 years	Pediatric hospital Pediatric hematology staff	Transition Pilot Program including a tour of adult SCD programs, lunch discussion with pediatric staff and scheduling of the first adult visit by the pediatric hematology case manager

Citation Location	Model	Population	Setting	Description
Chaturvedi et al., 2009[22] Australia **	**Transition program**	Pediatric kidney transplant recipients	Children's hospital renal clinic Transition coordinator, transition adult nephrologist, and transition nurse	Transition clinic, development of self-management skills and a written transition summary
Craig et al., 2007[23] Australia	**Transition program**	Youth with cystic fibrosis	Children's hospital	Phase-based transition program, including a preparation phase in early adolescence and an active phase that begins around age 16.
Byron and Madge, 2001[24]	**Transition Programme**	Youth with cystic fibrosis	Children's hospital	
Price et al., 2011[25] UK	**Transitions Pathway model**	Youth with type 1 diabetes aged 16-18 years	Hospital	Transitions Pathway model including 4 preparatory visits leading up to transfer to the 16 – 25 year old clinic focusing on fitting diabetes care into current and future life and ensuring that patients received adequate advice. Upon request, pediatrician attended first visit in the young adult clinic.
Gleeson et al., 2013[26] UK **	**Young Person Clinic**	Individuals with congenital adrenal hyperplasia	Children's hospital Pediatric and adult endocrine teams	Young Person Clinic (YPC) at which the youth is introduced to an adult endocrinologist
Bent et al., 2002[27] UK **	**Young Adult Teams**	Youth with long-term physical disability	4 regions	Young Adult Teams, including multidisciplinary teams including a consultant in rehabilitation medicine, a psychologist, therapists and a social worker

** also in the transition program evaluation table in GQ3

References for Appendix C.

1. A consensus statement on health care transitions for young adults with special health care needs. Pediatrics. 2002 Dec;110(6 Pt 2):1304-6. PMID: 12456949

2. Clayton PE, Cuneo RC, Juul A, et al. Consensus statement on the management of the GH-treated adolescent in the transition to adult care. Eur J Endocrinol. 2005 Feb;152(2):165-70. PMID: 15745921

3. Nutt DJ, Fone K, Asherson P, et al. Evidence-based guidelines for management of attention-deficit/hyperactivity disorder in adolescents in transition to adult services and in adults: recommendations from the British Association for Psychopharmacology. J Psychopharmacol. 2007 Jan;21(1):10-41. PMID: 17092962

4. Peters A, Laffel L. Diabetes care for emerging adults: recommendations for transition from pediatric to adult diabetes care systems: a position statement of the American Diabetes Association, with representation by the American College of Osteopathic Family Physicians, the American Academy of Pediatrics, the American Association of Clinical Endocrinologists, the American Osteopathic Association, the Centers for Disease Control and Prevention, Children with Diabetes, The Endocrine Society, the International Society for Pediatric and Adolescent Diabetes, Juvenile Diabetes Research Foundation International, the National Diabetes Education Program, and the Pediatric Endocrine Society (formerly Lawson Wilkins Pediatric Endocrine Society). Diabetes Care. 2011 Nov;34(11):2477-85. PMID: 22025785

5. Watson AR, Harden PN, Ferris ME, et al. Transition from pediatric to adult renal services: a consensus statement by the International Society of Nephrology (ISN) and the International Pediatric Nephrology Association (IPNA). Kidney Int. 2011 Oct;80(7):704-7. PMID: 21832978

6. Webb N, Harden P, Lewis C, et al. Building consensus on transition of transplant patients from paediatric to adult healthcare. Arch Dis Child. 2010 Aug;95(8):606-11. PMID: 20515964

7. Jurasek L, Ray L, Quigley D. Development and implementation of an adolescent epilepsy transition clinic. J Neurosci Nurs. 2010 Aug;42(4):181-9. PMID: 20804112

8. Transition from paediatric to adult endocrine care in patients with childhood onset growth hormone deficiency. J Pediatr Endocrinol Metab. 2004 Feb;17 Suppl 2:267-71. PMID: 15116950

9. Betz CL, Redcay G. Creating Healthy Futures: an innovative nurse-managed transition clinic for adolescents and young adults with special health care needs. Pediatr Nurs. 2003 Jan-Feb;29(1):25-30. PMID: 12630502

10. Amaria K, Stinson J, Cullen-Dean G, et al. Tools for addressing systems issues in transition. Healthc Q. 2011 Oct;14 Spec No 3:72-6. PMID: 22008577

11. Paone MC, Wigle M, Saewyc E. The ON TRAC model for transitional care of adolescents. Prog Transplant. 2006 Dec;16(4):291-302. PMID: 17183935

12. Kaufmann Rauen K, Sawin KJ, Bartelt T, et al. Transitioning adolescents and young adults with a chronic health condition to adult healthcare - an exemplar program. Rehabil Nurs. 2013 Mar-Apr;38(2):63-72. PMID: 23529944

13. Stewart D, Freeman M, Law M, et al. The best journey to adult life for youth with disabilities. An evidence-based model and best practice guidelines for the transition to adulthood. McMaster University, Hamilton Ontario: CanHealth Centre for Childhood Disability Research; 2009. http://transitions.canchild.ca/en/OurResearch/bestpractices.asp

14. Smith GM, Lewis VR, Whitworth E, et al. Growing up with sickle cell disease: a pilot study of a transition program for adolescents with sickle cell disease. J Pediatr Hematol Oncol. 2011 Jul;33(5):379-82. PMID: 21602723

15. Vanelli M, Caronna S, Adinolfi B, et al. Effectiveness of an uninterrupted procedure to transfer adolescents with Type 1 diabetes from the Paediatric to the Adult Clinic held in the same

hospital: eight-year experience with the Parma protocol. Diabetes Nutr Metab. 2004 Oct;17(5):304-8. PMID: 16295053

16. Chaudhry SR, Keaton M, Nasr SZ. Evaluation of a cystic fibrosis transition program from pediatric to adult care. Pediatr Pulmonol. 2013 Jul;48(7):658-65. PMID: 22888094

17. Gerber BS, Solomon MC, Shaffer TL, et al. Evaluation of an internet diabetes self-management training program for adolescents and young adults. Diabetes Technol Ther. 2007 Feb;9(1):60-7. PMID: 17316099

18. Maslow G, Adams C, Willis M, et al. An evaluation of a positive youth development program for adolescents with chronic illness. J Adolesc Health. 2013 Feb;52(2):179-85. PMID: 23332482

19. Van Walleghem N, MacDonald CA, Dean HJ. Building connections for young adults with type 1 diabetes mellitus in Manitoba: feasibility and acceptability of a transition initiative. Chronic Dis Can. 2006;27(3):130-4. PMID: 17306065

20. Van Walleghem N, Macdonald CA, Dean HJ. Evaluation of a systems navigator model for transition from pediatric to adult care for young adults with type 1 diabetes. Diabetes Care. 2008 Aug;31(8):1529-30. PMID: 18458141

21. Hankins JS, Osarogiagbon R, Adams-Graves P, et al. A transition pilot program for adolescents with sickle cell disease. J Pediatr Health Care. 2012 Nov-Dec;26(6):e45-9. PMID: 22819193

22. Chaturvedi S, Jones CL, Walker RG, et al. The transition of kidney transplant recipients: a work in progress. Pediatr Nephrol. 2009 May;24(5):1055-60. PMID: 19238453

23. Craig SL, Towns S, Bibby H. Moving on from paediatric to adult health care: an initial evaluation of a transition program for young people with cystic fibrosis. Int J Adolesc Med Health. 2007 Jul-Sep;19(3):333-43. PMID: 17937150

24. Bryon M, Madge S. Transition from paediatric to adult care: psychological principles. J R Soc Med. 2001;94 Suppl 40:5-7. PMID: 11601164

25. Price CS, Corbett S, Lewis-Barned N, et al. Implementing a transition pathway in diabetes: a qualitative study of the experiences and suggestions of young people with diabetes. Child Care Health Dev. 2011 Nov;37(6):852-60. PMID: 22007985

26. Gleeson H, Davis J, Jones J, et al. The challenge of delivering endocrine care and successful transition to adult services in adolescents with congenital adrenal hyperplasia: experience in a single centre over 18 years. Clin Endocrinol (Oxf). 2013 Jan;78(1):23-8. PMID: 23009615

27. Bent N, Tennant A, Swift T, et al. Team approach versus ad hoc health services for young people with physical disabilities: a retrospective cohort study. Lancet. 2002 Oct 26;360(9342):1280-6. PMID: 12414202

Appendix D. Reasons for Exclusion

Exclusion Code	Exclusion Reason	Count
X-1	Not youth	15
X-2	Population does not have a special health need	7
X-3	Publication did not address transition from pediatric to adult health care	110
X-4	Not a health care setting	30
X-5	Original research and does not address a guiding question	102
X-6	Not original research and does not address a guiding question	130
X-7	Unavailable	18
X-8	Duplicate	4

References

1. Program coordinates care, resources for medically complex children. Hosp Case Manag 2003 Oct;11(10):145-8. PMID: 13677693. *X-3, X-6*

2. Transition from paediatric to adult endocrine care in patients with childhood onset growth hormone deficiency. J Pediatr Endocrinol Metab 2004 Feb;17 Suppl 2:267-71. PMID: 15116950. *X-6*

3. Health assessments not holistic in transition. Learning Disability Practice 2004;7(2):6-. *X-6*

4. Few adolescents with special health care needs receive adequate transition from pediatric to adult-oriented health care. AHRQ Research Activities 2005(300):9-. *X-6*

5. Hospitalization patterns change as young people with congenital heart disease transition from adolescence to adulthood. AHRQ Research Activities 2007(323):4-. *X-3*

6. GAO report explores adult transition challenges for youth with SMI: bipartisan lawmakers introduce legislation to address barriers, provide grants. Mental Health Weekly 2008;18(26):1-3. *X-6*

7. From the American Academy of Pediatrics: Policy statements--Supplemental Security Income (SSI) for children and youth with disabilities. Pediatrics 2009 Dec;124(6):1702-8. PMID: 19948637. *X-3, X-4*

8. Project seeks replicable service model for youth in transition. Mental Health Weekly 2009;19(34):3-4. *X-6*

9. Clinical Report--Supporting the Health Care Transition From Adolescence to Adulthood in the Medical Home. Pediatrics 2011;128(1):182-200. PMID: 21708806. *X-8*

10. Abstracts. Adoption & Fostering 2013;37(4):426-9. *X-1, X-2, X-3*

11. Agwu AL, Fairlie L. Antiretroviral treatment, management challenges and outcomes in perinatally HIV-infected adolescents. J Int AIDS Soc 2013;16:18579. PMID: 23782477. *X-6*

12. Allen D. Into the abyss. Learning Disability Practice 2008;11(5):9. *X-6*

13. Allen D, Gregory J. The transition from children's to adult diabetes services: understanding the 'problem'. Diabet Med 2009 Feb;26(2):162-6. PMID: 19236619. *X-6*

14. Allison S, Baune BT, Roeger L, et al. Youth consultation-liaison psychiatry: how can we improve outcomes for young people with chronic illness? Aust N Z J Psychiatry. 2013 Jul;47(7):613-6. PMID: 23430841. *X-6*

15. Al-Yateem N. Child to adult: transitional care for young adults with cystic fibrosis. Br J Nurs 2012 Jul 26-Aug 8;21(14):850-4. PMID: 23252167. *X-2*

16. Amaria K, Stinson J, Cullen-Dean G, et al. Tools for addressing systems issues in transition. Healthc Q 2011 Oct;14 Spec No 3:72-6. PMID: 22008577. *X-6*

17. Andemariam B, Owarish-Gross J, Grady J, et al. Identification of risk factors for an unsuccessful transition from pediatric to adult sickle cell disease care. Pediatr Blood Cancer. 2014 Apr;61(4):697-701. PMID: 24347402. *X-8*

18. Annunziato RA, Shemesh E. Tackling the spectrum of transition: what can be done in pediatric settings? Pediatr Transplant 2010 Nov;14(7):820-2. PMID: 20946515. *X-6*

19. Arango P. Family-centered care. Acad Pediatr 2011 Mar-Apr;11(2):97-9. PMID: 21282085. *X-3*

20. Arcelus J, Cashmore R. Child to adult: managing the transition. British Journal of Healthcare Management 2008:9-14. *X-6*

21. Archbold S. Children with cochlear implants--what is needed--and what is wanted in the long-term? Cochlear Implants Int 2010 Jun;11 Suppl 1:225-7. PMID: 21756618. *X-3*

22. Baines JM. Promoting better care: transition from child to adult services. Nurs Stand 2009 Jan 14-20;23(19):35-40. PMID: 19326623. *X-6*

23. Barendse RM, aan de Kerk DJ, Kindermann A, et al. Transition of adolescents with inflammatory bowel disease from pediatric to adult care: A survey of Dutch adult gastroenterologists' perspectives. International Journal of Child and Adolescent Health 2010 2012-09-10;3(4):609-16. *X-7*

24. Bates K, Bartoshesky L, Friedland A. As the child with chronic disease grows up: transitioning adolescents with special health care needs to adult-centered health care. Del Med J 2003 Jun;75(6):217-20. PMID: 12929331. *X-6*

25. Beacham BL, Deatrick JA. Health care autonomy in children with chronic conditions: implications for self-care and family management. Nurs Clin North Am 2013 Jun;48(2):305-17. PMID: 23659815. *X-3, X-6*

26. Beattie RM. Symposium 6: Young people, artificial nutrition and transitional care: Nutrition, growth and puberty in children and adolescents with Crohn's disease. Proc Nutr Soc 2010 Feb;69(1):174-7. PMID: 19968909. *X-6*

27. Begley T. Transition to adult care for young people with long-term conditions. Br J Nurs 2013 May 9-22;22(9):506, 8-11. PMID: 23752622. *X-5*

28. Bell LE, Bartosh SM, Davis CL, et al. Adolescent Transition to Adult Care in Solid Organ Transplantation: a consensus conference report. Am J Transplant 2008 Nov;8(11):2230-42. PMID: 18822088. *X-6*

29. Benden C. Specific aspects of children and adolescents undergoing lung transplantation. Curr Opin Organ Transplant 2012 Oct;17(5):509-14. PMID: 22941318. *X-3*

30. Berge JM, Patterson JM, Goetz D, et al. Gender differences in young adults' perceptions of living with cystic fibrosis during the transition to adulthood: a qualitative investigation. Families, Systems & Health: The Journal of Collaborative Family HealthCare 2007;25(2):190-203. *X-5*

31. Betz CL. Health care transitions of youth with special health care needs: the never ending journey. Commun Nurs Res 2008 Spring;41:13-29. PMID: 18822668. *X-6*

32. Betz CL, Linroth R, Butler C, et al. Spina bifida: what we learned from consumers. Pediatr Clin North Am 2010 Aug;57(4):935-44. PMID: 20883883. *X-5*

33. Betz CL, Smith K. Measuring health care transition planning outcomes: Challenges and issues. International Journal of Child and Adolescent Health 2010 2012-09-10;3(4):463-72. *X-7*

34. Bhat AH, Sahn DJ. Congenital heart disease never goes away, even when it has been 'treated': the adult with congenital heart disease. Curr Opin Pediatr 2004 Oct;16(5):500-7. PMID: 15367842. *X-6*

35. Bhatia S, Ahmad F, Miller I, et al. Surgical treatment of refractory status epilepticus in children: clinical article. J Neurosurg Pediatr 2013 Oct;12(4):360-6. PMID: 23971636. *X-3*

36. Bickman L, Lambert EW, Andrade AR, et al. The Fort Bragg continuum of care for children and adolescents: mental health outcomes over 5 years. J Consult Clin Psychol 2000 Aug;68(4):710-6. PMID: 10965645. *X-3*

37. Bindels-de Heus KG, van Staa A, van Vliet I, et al. Transferring young people with profound intellectual and multiple disabilities from pediatric to adult medical care: parents' experiences and recommendations. Intellect Dev Disabil. 2013 Jun;51(3):176-89. PMID: 23834214. *X-1*

38. Blackman JA, Conaway MR. Adolescents With Cerebral Palsy: Transitioning to Adult Health Care Services. Clin Pediatr (Phila) 2013 Nov 25PMID: 24275216. *X-5*

39. Blomquist KB. Healthy and ready to work--Kentucky: incorporating transition into a state program for children with special health care needs. Pediatr Nurs 2006 Nov-Dec;32(6):515-28. PMID: 17256289. *X-6*

40. Blomquist KB. Health, education, work, and independence of young adults with disabilities. Orthop Nurs 2006 May-Jun;25(3):168-87. PMID: 16735848. *X-5*

41. Blum RW. Introduction. Improving transition for adolescents with special health care needs from pediatric to adult-centered health care. Pediatrics 2002 Dec;110(6 Pt 2):1301-3. PMID: 12456948. *X-6*

42. Brennan LJ, Rolfe PM. Transition from pediatric to adult health services: the perioperative care perspective. Paediatr Anaesth 2011 Jun;21(6):630-5. PMID: 21414078. *X-6*

43. Broadhurst S, Yates K, Mullen B. An evaluation of the My Way transition programme. Tizard Learning Disability Review 2012;17(3):124-34. *X-4*

44. Brodie L, Crisp J, McCormack B, et al. Journeying from nirvana with mega-mums and broken hearts: The complex dynamics of transition

from paediatric to adult settings. International Journal of Child and Adolescent Health 2010 2012-09-10;3(4):517-26. *X-7*

45. Brooks F, Bunn F, Morgan J. Transition for adolescents with long-term conditions: event to process. Br J Community Nurs 2009 Jul;14(7):301-4. PMID: 19597382. *X-6*

46. Bruder MB. The role of the physician in early intervention for children with developmental disabilities. Conn Med 2004 Sep;68(8):507-14. PMID: 15468622. *X-3*

47. Bucuvalas JC, Alonso E, Magee JC, et al. Improving long-term outcomes after liver transplantation in children. Am J Transplant 2008 Dec;8(12):2506-13. PMID: 18853949. *X-3*

48. Burke R, Liptak GS. Providing a primary care medical home for children and youth with spina bifida. Pediatrics 2011 Dec;128(6):e1645-57. PMID: 22123894. *X-3*

49. Burke SD. Diabetes in transition: Factors affecting diabetes self-management in college students: University of Illinois at Chicago, Health Sciences Center; 2004. *X-5*

50. Burns JJ, Sadof M, Kamat D. The adolescent with a chronic illness. Pediatr Ann 2006 Mar;35(3):206-10, 14-6. PMID: 16570487. *X-6*

51. Busse FP, Hiermann P, Galler A, et al. Evaluation of patients' opinion and metabolic control after transfer of young adults with type 1 diabetes from a pediatric diabetes clinic to adult care. Horm Res 2007;67(3):132-8. PMID: 17065819. *X-5*

52. Camacho CB, Hemmeter J. Linking youth transition support services: results from two demonstration projects. Soc Secur Bull 2013;73(1):59-71. PMID: 23687742. *X-4*

53. Camfield P, Camfield C. Transition to adult care for children with chronic neurological disorders. Ann Neurol 2011 Mar;69(3):437-44. PMID: 21391239. *X-6*

54. Carroll AE, DiMeglio LA, Stein S, et al. Contracting and monitoring relationships for adolescents with type 1 diabetes: a pilot study. Diabetes Technol Ther 2011 May;13(5):543-9. PMID: 21406011. *X-3*

55. Cheak-Zamora NC, Yang X, Farmer JE, et al. Disparities in transition planning for youth with autism spectrum disorder. Pediatrics 2013 Mar;131(3):447-54. PMID: 23400613. *X-5*

56. Chi DL. Medical Care Transition Planning and Dental Care Use for Youth with Special Health Care Needs During the Transition from Adolescence to Young Adulthood: A Preliminary Explanatory Model. Matern Child Health J 2013 Jun 28PMID: 23812799. *X-5*

57. Chira P, Nugent L, Miller K, et al. Living Profiles: design of a health media platform for teens with special healthcare needs. J Biomed Inform 2010 Oct;43(5 Suppl):S9-12. PMID: 20937487. *X-6*

58. Chisanga E. Applying specialist nurse skills to improve epilepsy adolescent transition services. British Journal of Neuroscience Nursing 2009;5(6):274-7. *X-7*

59. Christian CW, Schwarz DF. Child maltreatment and the transition to adult-based medical and mental health care. Pediatrics 2011 Jan;127(1):139-45. PMID: 21149424. *X-4*

60. Christie CD, Pierre RB. Eliminating vertically-transmitted HIV/AIDS while improving access to treatment and care for women, children and adolescents in Jamaica. West Indian Med J 2012 Jul;61(4):396-404. PMID: 23240475. *X-3*

61. Clark HB, Koroloff N, Geller J, et al. Research on transition to adulthood: building the evidence base to inform services and supports for youth and young adults with serious mental health disorders. J Behav Health Serv Res 2008 Oct;35(4):365-72. PMID: 18726695. *X-6*

62. Clayton PE, Cuneo RC, Juul A, et al. Consensus statement on the management of the GH-treated adolescent in the transition to adult care. Eur J Endocrinol 2005 Feb;152(2):165-70. PMID: 15745921. *X-6*

63. Cohen E, Berry JG, Camacho X, et al. Patterns and costs of health care use of children with medical complexity. Pediatrics 2012 Dec;130(6):e1463-70. PMID: 23184117. *X-3*

64. Colver AF, Merrick H, Deverill M, et al. Study protocol: Longitudinal study of the transition of young people with complex health needs from child to adult health services. BMC Public Health 2013 Jul 23;13(1):675. PMID: 23875722. *X-6*

65. Conway GS. Congenital adrenal hyperplasia: adolescence and transition. Horm Res 2007;68 Suppl 5:155-7. PMID: 18174736. *X-6*

66. Cooley WC. Providing a primary care medical home for children and youth with cerebral palsy. Pediatrics 2004 Oct;114(4):1106-13. PMID: 15466117. *X-3*

67. Couriel J. Asthma in adolescence. Paediatr Respir Rev 2003 Mar;4(1):47-54. PMID: 12615032. *X-5*

68. Cox S. Age-appropriate care. Nurs Stand 2011 Jan 19-25;25(20):23. PMID: 21329167. *X-6*

69. Craig SL, Towns S, Bibby H. Moving on from paediatric to adult health care: an initial evaluation of a transition program for young people with cystic fibrosis. Int J Adolesc Med Health 2007 Jul-Sep;19(3):333-43. PMID: 17937150. *X-5*

70. Cramm JM, Strating MM, Sonneveld HM, et al. The Longitudinal Relationship Between Satisfaction with Transitional Care and Social and Emotional Quality of Life Among Chronically Ill Adolescents. Appl Res Qual Life 2013;8:481-91. PMID: 24058386. *X-5*

71. Creighton SM, Wood D. Complex gynaecological and urological problems in adolescents: challenges and transition. Postgrad Med J 2013 Jan;89(1047):34-8. PMID: 23043130. *X-3*

72. Crosier J, Wise LC. Coming of age. Cystic fibrosis--once a childhood disease--makes its way to adulthood. Nurs Manage 2001 Nov;32(11):30-1. PMID: 15129541. *X-6*

73. Cross KP, Santucci KA. Transitional medicine: will emergency medicine physicians be ready for the growing population of adults with congenital heart disease? Pediatr Emerg Care 2006 Dec;22(12):775-81. PMID: 17198208. *X-1*

74. Cuttell K, Hilton D, Drew J. Preparation for transition to adult diabetes services. Paediatr Nurs 2005 Mar;17(2):28-30. PMID: 15793986. *X-4*

75. Daily DK, Ardinger HH, Holmes GE. Identification and evaluation of mental retardation. Am Fam Physician 2000 Feb 15;61(4):1059-67, 70. PMID: 10706158. *X-3*

76. Daly B, Kral MC, Tarazi RA. The role of neuropsychological evaluation in pediatric sickle cell disease. Clin Neuropsychol 2011 Aug;25(6):903-25. PMID: 21563016. *X-3*

77. Daneman D, Nakhla M. Moving On: Transition of Teens With Type 1 Diabetes to Adult Care. Diabetes Spectrum 2011 2011 Winter;24(1):14-8. *X-6*

78. Davies MC. Lost in transition: the needs of adolescents with Turner syndrome. BJOG 2010 Jan;117(2):134-6. PMID: 20002393. *X-6*

79. Davies PS, Rupp K. An overview of the National Survey of SSI Children and Families and related products. Soc Secur Bull 2005;66(2):7-20. PMID: 16878425. *X-3*

80. Davis E, Barnhill LJ, Saeed SA. Treatment models for treating patients with combined mental illness and developmental disability. Psychiatr Q 2008 Sep;79(3):205-23. PMID: 18726155. *X-3*

81. Davis JT. Thoughts from the transition zone. N Engl J Med 2006 Jul 20;355(3):235-6. PMID: 16855262. *X-3*

82. Davis M, Koroloff N, Johnsen M. Social network analysis of child and adult interorganizational connections. Psychiatr Rehabil J 2012 Winter;35(3):265-72. PMID: 22246126. *X-4, X-5*

83. De Sanctis V, Soliman A, Mohamed Y. Reproductive health in young male adults with chronic diseases in childhood. Pediatr Endocrinol Rev 2013 Mar-Apr;10(3):284-96. PMID: 23724436. *X-3*

84. DeBell D, Carter R. Impact of transition on public health in Ukraine: case study of the HIV/AIDS epidemic. BMJ 2005 Jul 23;331(7510):216-9. PMID: 16037461. *X-4*

85. Dellon ES, Jones PD, Martin NB, et al. Health-care transition from pediatric to adult-focused gastroenterology in patients with eosinophilic esophagitis. Dis Esophagus 2013 Jan;26(1):7-13. PMID: 22309247. *X-6*

86. Dicianno BE, Fairman AD, Juengst SB, et al. Using the spina bifida life course model in clinical practice: an interdisciplinary approach. Pediatr Clin North Am 2010 Aug;57(4):945-57. PMID: 20883884. *X-6*

87. Dimitropoulos G, Tran AF, Agarwal P, et al. Challenges in making the transition between pediatric and adult eating disorder programs: a qualitative study from the perspective of service providers. Eat Disord 2013;21(1):1-15. PMID: 23241086. *X-5*

88. Donkervoort M, Wiegerink DJ, van Meeteren J, et al. Transition to adulthood: validation of the Rotterdam Transition Profile for young adults with cerebral palsy and normal intelligence. Dev Med Child Neurol 2009 Jan;51(1):53-62. PMID: 19021680. *X-4*

89. Douglass LM. Introduction: Transitioning care for adults with Lennox-Gastaut syndrome: challenges and promises. Epilepsia 2011 Aug;52 Suppl 5:1-2. PMID: 21790559. *X-6*

90. Doyle LW, Anderson PJ. Adult outcome of extremely preterm infants. Pediatrics 2010 Aug;126(2):342-51. PMID: 20679313. *X-3*

91. Doyle M, Siegel R, Supe K. Stages of change and transitioning for adolescent patients with obesity and hypertension. Adv Chronic Kidney Dis 2006 Oct;13(4):386-93. PMID: 17045224. *X-6*

92. Drell M. Innovations: Child & adolescent psychiatry: "Sweet are the uses of adversity": a transition program for children discharged from an inpatient unit. Psychiatr Serv 2006 Jan;57(1):31-3. PMID: 16403727. *X-3*

93. Dudman L, Rapley P, Wilson S. Development of a transition readiness scale for young adults with cystic fibrosis: face and conten validity. Neonatal, Paediatric & Child Health Nursing 2011;14(2):9-13. *X-5*

94. Dugueperoux I, Tamalet A, Sermet-Gaudelus I, et al. Clinical changes of patients with cystic fibrosis during transition from pediatric to adult care. J Adolesc Health 2008 Nov;43(5):459-65. PMID: 18848674. *X-5*

95. Dupuis F. Modelisation systemique de la transition pour des familles ayant un adolescent atteint de fibrose kystique en phase pre-transfert vers l'establissement adulte: Universite de Montreal (Canada); 2007. *X-7*

96. Dupuis F, Duhamel F, Gendron S. Transitioning care of an adolescent with cystic fibrosis: development of systemic hypothesis between parents, adolescents, and health care professionals. J Fam Nurs 2011 Aug;17(3):291-311. PMID: 21813812. *X-3*

97. Ellingford C. Short report: refocusing transition clinics. Paediatr Nurs 2006 Jul;18(6):37. PMID: 16881503. *X-6*

98. Evans J, McDougall J, Baldwin P. An evaluation of the "Youth en Route" program. Phys Occup Ther Pediatr 2006;26(4):63-87. PMID: 17135070. *X-4*

99. Fair CD, Sullivan K, Dizney R, et al. "It's like losing a part of my family": transition expectations of adolescents living with perinatally acquired HIV and their guardians. AIDS Patient Care STDS 2012 Jul;26(7):423-9. PMID: 22686235. *X-5*

100. Fair CD, Sullivan K, Gatto A. Indicators of transition success for youth living with HIV: perspectives of pediatric and adult infectious disease care providers. AIDS Care 2011 Aug;23(8):965-70. PMID: 21390882. *X-5*

101. Fegran L, C, Uhrenfeldt L, et al. Adolescents' and young adults' transition experiences when transferring from paediatric to adult care: A qualitative metasynthesis. International Journal of Nursing Studies 2014;51(1):123-35. PMID: 23490470. *X-6*

102. Fernandes SM, Landzberg MJ, Fishman LN, et al. Clinician perceptions of transition of patients with pediatric-onset chronic disease to adult medical care: Comparing a pediatric facility integrated within an adult institution with a free-standing pediatric hospital. International Journal of Child and Adolescent Health 2012 2013-04-09;5(3):281-9. PMID: 1324548491; 2013-05161-005. *X-7*

103. Ferris ME, Ferris MT, Viall C, et al. The self-management and transition to adulthood program "UNC STARX": Instruments and lessons from the field. International Journal of Child and Adolescent Health 2013 2013-10-17;6(2):137-47. PMID: 1440033862; 2013-27562-002. *X-7*

104. Ferris ME, Harward DH, Bickford K, et al. A clinical tool to measure the components of health-care transition from pediatric care to adult care: the UNC TR(x)ANSITION scale. Ren Fail 2012;34(6):744-53. PMID: 22583152. *X-5*

105. Ferris ME, Wood D, Ferris MT, et al. Toward evidence-based health care transition: The Health Care Transition Research Consortium. Int J Child Adolesc Health 2010;3(4):479-86. *X-6*

106. Ferro MA. Adolescents and young adults with physical illness: a comparative study of psychological distress. Acta Paediatr 2014 Jan;103(1):e32-7. PMID: 24117721. *X-3*

107. Flume PA, Anderson DL, Hardy KK, et al. Transition programs in cystic fibrosis centers: perceptions of pediatric and adult program directors. Pediatr Pulmonol 2001 Jun;31(6):443-50. PMID: 11389577. *X-5*

108. Forcier M, Ahlm S, Boudos R, et al. A hospital-wide initiative to support medically complex adolescents and young adult's transition experience: The process of a systems approach to transition in a tertiary care setting. International Journal of Child and Adolescent Health 2010 2012-09-10;3(4):561-74. *X-7*

109. Forsyth RJ, Kelly TP, Wicks B, et al. 'Must try harder?': a family empowerment intervention for acquired brain injury. Pediatr Rehabil 2005 Apr-Jun;8(2):140-3. PMID: 16089254. *X-3*

110. Foster C, Waelbrouck A, Peltier A. Adolescents and HIV infection. Curr Opin HIV AIDS 2007 Sep;2(5):431-6. PMID: 19372923. *X-6*

111. Fredericks EM, Dore-Stites D, Well A, et al. Assessment of transition readiness skills and adherence in pediatric liver transplant recipients. Pediatr Transplant 2010 Dec;14(8):944-53. PMID: 20598086. *X-5*

112. Freed GL, Hudson EJ. Transitioning children with chronic diseases to adult care: current knowledge, practices, and directions. J Pediatr 2006 Jun;148(6):824-7. PMID: 16769396. *X-6*

113. Friedman S, Chen C, Chapman JS, et al. Neurodevelopmental outcomes of congenital diaphragmatic hernia survivors followed in a multidisciplinary clinic at ages 1 and 3. J Pediatr Surg 2008 Jun;43(6):1035-43. PMID: 18558179. *X-3*

114. Frimberger D, Cheng E, Kropp BP. The current management of the neurogenic bladder in children with spina bifida. Pediatr Clin North Am 2012 Aug;59(4):757-67. PMID: 22857827. *X-3*

115. Frisch D, Msall ME. Health, functioning, and participation of adolescents and adults with cerebral palsy: a review of outcomes research. Dev Disabil Res Rev. 2013 Aug;18(1):84-94. PMID: 23949832.*X-3, X-4*

116. Gall C, Kingsnorth S, Healy H. Growing up ready: a shared management approach. Phys Occup Ther Pediatr 2006;26(4):47-62. PMID: 17135069. *X-4*

117. Garvey KC, Finkelstein JA, Laffel LM, et al. Transition experiences and health care utilization among young adults with type 1 diabetes. Patient Prefer Adherence 2013;7:761-9. PMID: 23990711. *X-5*

118. Geerts E, van de Wiel H, Tamminga R. A pilot study on the effects of the transition of paediatric to adult health care in patients with haemophilia and in their parents: patient and parent worries, parental illness-related distress and health-related Quality of Life. Haemophilia 2008 Sep;14(5):1007-13. PMID: 18624704. *X-3*

119. Gelder C. Care of adolescents in transition. Practice Nursing 2009;20(9):444-8. *X-3*

120. Gilmer TP, Ojeda VD, Fawley-King K, et al. Change in mental health service use after offering youth-specific versus adult programs to transition-age youths. Psychiatr Serv 2012 Jun;63(6):592-6. PMID: 22422015. *X-5*

121. Glader LJ, Palfrey JS. Care of the child assisted by technology. Pediatr Rev 2009 Nov;30(11):439-44; quiz 45. PMID: 19884284. *X-3*

122. Goldstein SL, Gerson AC, Goldman CW, et al. Quality of life for children with chronic kidney disease. Semin Nephrol 2006 Mar;26(2):114-7. PMID: 16530604. *X-3*

123. Goldstone AP, Holland AJ, Hauffa BP, et al. Recommendations for the diagnosis and management of Prader-Willi syndrome. J Clin Endocrinol Metab 2008 Nov;93(11):4183-97. PMID: 18697869. *X-6*

124. Gupta P. Caring for a teen with congenital heart disease. Pediatr Clin North Am 2014 Feb;61(1):207-28. PMID: 24267466. *X-6*

125. Gurvitz MZ, Inkelas M, Lee M, et al. Changes in hospitalization patterns among patients with congenital heart disease during the transition from adolescence to adulthood. J Am Coll Cardiol 2007 Feb 27;49(8):875-82. PMID: 17320746. *X-3, X-5*

126. Haber MG, Karpur A, Deschenes N, et al. Predicting improvement of transitioning young

people in the partnerships for youth transition initiative: findings from a multisite demonstration. J Behav Health Serv Res 2008 Oct;35(4):488-513. PMID: 18636333. *X-4*

127. Hagenfeldt KB. Congenital adrenal hyperplasia due to 21-hydroxylase deficiency--the adult woman. Growth Horm IGF Res 2004 Jun;14 Suppl A:S67-71. PMID: 15135781. *X-3*

128. Hall J, Starrett B. Assessing the health care needs of Kansas' young adults with disabilities. Kans Nurse 2007 Aug;82(7):5-7. PMID: 17902555. *X-3, X-5*

129. Hamdani Y, Jetha A, Norman C. Systems thinking perspectives applied to healthcare transition for youth with disabilities: a paradigm shift for practice, policy and research. Child Care Health Dev 2011 Nov;37(6):806-14. PMID: 22007980. *X-6*

130. Hanna KM. A framework for the youth with type 1 diabetes during the emerging adulthood transition. Nurs Outlook 2012 Nov-Dec;60(6):401-10. PMID: 22226223. *X-6*

131. Harden PN, Nadine P. Pediatric to adult transition: a personal experience. Prog Transplant 2006 Dec;16(4):324-8. PMID: 17183939. *X-6*

132. Harris D. Children with complex needs are overlooked in transition... Art & science, January 14. Nursing Standard 2009;23(21):32-3. *X-3*

133. Harris KM, Gordon-Larsen P, Chantala K, et al. Longitudinal trends in race/ethnic disparities in leading health indicators from adolescence to young adulthood. Arch Pediatr Adolesc Med 2006 Jan;160(1):74-81. PMID: 16389215. *X-3*

134. Heflinger CA, Hoffman C. Transition age youth in publicly funded systems: identifying high-risk youth for policy planning and improved service delivery. J Behav Health Serv Res 2008 Oct;35(4):390-401. PMID: 17187298. *X-4*

135. Helgeson VS, Palladino DK, Reynolds KA, et al. Relationships and Health Among Emerging Adults With and Without Type 1 Diabetes. Health Psychol 2013 Aug 5PMID: 23914816. *X-3*

136. Hellstedt LF. Transitional care issues influencing access to health care: employability and insurability. Nurs Clin North Am 2004 Dec;39(4):741-53. PMID: 15561157. *X-4*

137. Hemker BG, Brousseau DC, Yan K, et al. When children with sickle-cell disease become adults: lack of outpatient care leads to increased use of the emergency department. Am J Hematol 2011 Oct;86(10):863-5. PMID: 21815184. *X-3*

138. Hergenroeder AC. The transition into adulthood for children and youth with special health care needs. Tex Med 2002 Feb;98(2):51-8. PMID: 11862893. *X-6*

139. Hersh A, von Scheven E, Yelin E. Adult outcomes of childhood-onset rheumatic diseases. Nat Rev Rheumatol 2011 May;7(5):290-5. PMID: 21487383. *X-5*

140. Hewer SC, Tyrrell J. Cystic fibrosis and the transition to adult health services. Arch Dis Child 2008 Oct;93(10):817-21. PMID: 18809702. *X-6*

141. Hilderson D, Corstjens F, Moons P, et al. Adolescents with juvenile idiopathic arthritis: who cares after the age of 16? Clin Exp Rheumatol 2010 Sep-Oct;28(5):790-7. PMID: 20863450. *X-5*

142. Hilderson D, Eyckmans L, Van der Elst K, et al. Transfer from paediatric rheumatology to the adult rheumatology setting: experiences and expectations of young adults with juvenile idiopathic arthritis. Clin Rheumatol. 2013 May;32(5):575-83. PMID: 23238606. *X-5*

143. Hilderson D, Saidi AS, Van Deyk K, et al. Attitude toward and current practice of transfer and transition of adolescents with congenital heart disease in the United States of America and Europe. Pediatr Cardiol 2009 Aug;30(6):786-93. PMID: 19365651. *X-5*

144. Hilderson D, Westhovens R, Wouters C, et al. Rationale, design and baseline data of a mixed methods study examining the clinical impact of a brief transition programme for young people with juvenile idiopathic arthritis: the DON'T RETARD project. BMJ Open 2013;3(12):e003591. PMID: 24302502. *X-5*

145. Hilliard ME, Perlus JG, Clark LM, et al. Perspectives from Before and After the Pediatric to Adult Care Transition: A Mixed-Methods Study in Type 1 Diabetes. Diabetes Care 2013 Oct 2PMID: 24089544. *X-5*

146. Hink H, Schellhase D. Transitioning families to adult cystic fibrosis care. J Spec Pediatr Nurs 2006 Oct;11(4):260-3. PMID: 16999750. *X-6*

147. Hodson ME. Treatment of cystic fibrosis in the adult. Respiration 2000;67(6):595-607. PMID: 11124641. *X-6*

148. Hoek W, Marko M, Fogel J, et al. Randomized controlled trial of primary care physician motivational interviewing versus brief advice to engage adolescents with an Internet-based depression prevention intervention: 6-month outcomes and predictors of improvement. Transl Res 2011 Dec;158(6):315-25. PMID: 22061038. *X-3*

149. Homer CJ, Cooley WC, Strickland B. Medical home 2009: what it is, where we were, and where we are today. Pediatr Ann 2009 Sep;38(9):483-90. PMID: 19772234. *X-3*

150. Hong DS. Child and adolescent psychiatrists are often tasked with the challenge of treating patients in various contexts. J Am Acad Child Adolesc Psychiatry. 2013 Sep;52(9):885-6. PMID: 23972687. *X-6*

151. Hosie P, Mair R. Primary Care 2011. J Fam Health Care 2011 Jul-Aug;21(4):38-41. PMID: 21980695. *X-2, X-3*

152. Hovish K, Weaver T, Islam Z, et al. Transition experiences of mental health service users, parents, and professionals in the United Kingdom: a qualitative study. Psychiatr Rehabil J 2012 Winter;35(3):251-7. PMID: 22246124. *X-5*

153. Hower H, Case BG, Hoeppner B, et al. Use of mental health services in transition age youth with bipolar disorder. J Psychiatr Pract 2013 Nov;19(6):464-76. PMID: 24241500. *X-5*

154. Hughes IA. Congenital adrenal hyperplasia: transitional care. Growth Horm IGF Res 2004 Jun;14 Suppl A:S60-6. PMID: 15135780. *X-6*

155. Hullmann SE, Chalmers LJ, Wisniewski AB. Transition from pediatric to adult care for adolescents and young adults with a disorder of sex development. J Pediatr Adolesc Gynecol 2012 Apr;25(2):155-7. PMID: 22530227. *X-6*

156. Hummel TZ, Tak E, Maurice-Stam H, et al. Psychosocial developmental trajectory of adolescents with inflammatory bowel disease. J Pediatr Gastroenterol Nutr. 2013 Aug;57(2):219-24. PMID: 23880627. *X-3*

157. Hunt S, Sharma N. Pediatric to adult-care transitions in childhood-onset chronic disease: hospitalist perspectives. J Hosp Med 2013 Nov;8(11):627-30. PMID: 24124077. *X-1*

158. Iannelli-Madigan G. Transitioning the adolescent with type 1 diabetes mellitus. J Pediatr Nurs 2012 Oct;27(5):602-4. PMID: 22819877. *X-6*

159. Iles N, Lowton K. Young people with cystic fibrosis' concerns for their future: when and how should concerns be addressed, and by whom? J Interprof Care 2008 Aug;22(4):436-8. PMID: 18800285. *X-5*

160. Iles N, Lowton K. What is the perceived nature of parental care and support for young people with cystic fibrosis as they enter adult health services? Health Soc Care Community 2010 Jan;18(1):21-9. PMID: 19637994. *X-4, X-5*

161. Irvine T, Srinivasan R, Casson DH, et al. Assessing the value of a pre-transfer meeting in IBD transition services. Gastrointestinal Nursing 2010;8(7):19. *X-5*

162. Ishizaki Y, Maru M, Higashino H, et al. The transition of adult patients with childhood-onset chronic diseases from pediatric to adult healthcare systems: a survey of the perceptions of Japanese pediatricians and child health nurses. Biopsychosoc Med 2012;6:8. PMID: 22433283. *X-5*

163. Iyer A, Appleton R. Transitional services for adolescents with epilepsy in the U.K.: a survey. Seizure 2013 Jul;22(6):433-7. PMID: 23498777. *X-5*

164. Jackett JM. Transition and beyond for individuals with autism spectrum disorders (ASD): a New Jersey case study of the adult service sector, its inherent shortcomings, and hope for the future. Seton Hall Law Rev 2010;40(4):1733-74. PMID: 21280391. *X-3, X-4*

165. Jackson KE. 157. Health Care Transition Guidance For Youth With Cerebral Palsy:An Analysis Of The National Survey Of Children With Special Health Care Needs. Journal of Adolescent Health 2012;50(2):S88-9. *X-5*

166. Jedeloo S, van Staa A, Latour JM, et al. Preferences for health care and self-management among Dutch adolescents with chronic conditions: a Q-methodological investigation. Int J Nurs Stud 2010 May;47(5):593-603. PMID: 19900675. *X-3*

167. Jermyn V. "You can't stay here!" Transition from paediatric to adult health care management for

liver transplant recipients. Transplant Journal of Australasia. 2013;22(3):15-8. PMID: 2012407304. *X-7*

168. Jones BL, Parker-Raley J, Barczyk A. Adolescent cancer survivors: identity paradox and the need to belong. Qual Health Res 2011 Aug;21(8):1033-40. PMID: 21447805. *X-2*

169. Jones SE, Hamilton S. The missing link: paediatric to adult transition in diabetes services. Br J Nurs 2008 Jul 10-23;17(13):842-7. PMID: 18856147. *X-6*

170. Jorgensen S. Lost in transition. Learning Disability Practice 2008;11(7):30-1. *X-6*

171. Kane DJ, Zotti ME, Rosenberg D. Factors associated with health care access for Mississippi children with special health care needs. Matern Child Health J 2005 Jun;9(2 Suppl):S23-31. PMID: 15973475. *X-3*

172. Karan OC, DonAroma P, Bruder MB, et al. Transitional assessment model for students with severe and/or multiple disabilities: competency-based community assessment. Intellect Dev Disabil 2010 Oct;48(5):387-92. PMID: 20973701. *X-3, X-4, X-6*

173. Karas DJ, Costain G, Chow EW, et al. Perceived burden and neuropsychiatric morbidities in adults with 22q11.2 deletion syndrome. J Intellect Disabil Res 2014 Feb;58(2):198-210. PMID: 23106770. *X-1*

174. Kaufman M. Role of adolescent development in the transition process. Prog Transplant 2006 Dec;16(4):286-90. PMID: 17183934. *X-4*

175. Kaufman M. Transition of cognitively delayed adolescent organ transplant recipients to adult care. Pediatr Transplant 2006 Jun;10(4):413-7. PMID: 16712597. *X-6*

176. Kennedy A, Sawyer S. Transition from pediatric to adult services: are we getting it right? Curr Opin Pediatr 2008 Aug;20(4):403-9. PMID: 18622194. *X-6*

177. Khan A, Baheerathan A, Hussain N, et al. Transition of children with epilepsies to adult care. Acta Paediatr 2013 Mar;102(3):216-21. PMID: 23190350. *X-6*

178. Kime N. 'Join us on our journey': exploring the experiences of children and young people with type 1 diabetes and their parents. Practical Diabetes. 2014;31(1):24-8. PMID: 2012448457. *X-5*

179. Kingsnorth S, Gall C, Beayni S, et al. Parents as transition experts? Qualitative findings from a pilot parent-led peer support group. Child Care Health Dev 2011 Nov;37(6):833-40. PMID: 22007983. *X-1*

180. Kirk S. Transitions in the lives of young people with complex healthcare needs. Child Care Health Dev 2008 Sep;34(5):567-75. PMID: 18796049. *X-5*

181. Kirkpatrick JN, Kim YY, Kaufman BD. Ethics priorities in adult congenital heart disease. Prog Cardiovasc Dis 2012 Nov-Dec;55(3):266-73 e3. PMID: 23217430. *X-6*

182. Klaas S, Hickey K. Transition to adult care. SCI Nurs 2001 Fall;18(3):158-60. PMID: 12503463. *X-6*

183. Knapp C, Huang IC, Hinojosa M, et al. Assessing the congruence of transition preparedness as reported by parents and their adolescents with special health care needs. Matern Child Health J 2013 Feb;17(2):352-8. PMID: 22415813. *X-5*

184. Ko B, McEnery G. The needs of physically disabled young people during transition to adult services. Child Care Health Dev 2004 Jul;30(4):317-23. PMID: 15191421. *X-5*

185. Kollipara S, Kaufman FR. Transition of diabetes care from pediatrics to adulthood. School Nurse News 2008 Jan;25(1):27-9. PMID: 18236837. *X-6*

186. Kossoff EH, Henry BJ, Cervenka MC. Transitioning pediatric patients receiving ketogenic diets for epilepsy into adulthood. Seizure 2013 Jul;22(6):487-9. PMID: 23571095. *X-5*

187. Kripke C, Giammona M, Fox A, et al. The CART model: Organized systems of care for transition age youth and adults with developmental disabilities. Int J Child Adolesc Health 2010;3(4):473-7. *X-6*

188. Kruse B, Riepe FG, Krone N, et al. Congenital adrenal hyperplasia - how to improve the transition from adolescence to adult life. Exp Clin Endocrinol Diabetes 2004 Jul;112(7):343-55. PMID: 15239019. *X-6*

189. Kuchenbuch M, Chemaly N, Chiron C, et al. Transition and transfer from pediatric to adult health care in epilepsy: a families' survey on Dravet syndrome. Epilepsy Behav 2013 Oct;29(1):161-5. PMID: 23973640. *X-5*

190. Ladores S. An evolutionary concept analysis of healthcare transition among adolescents with chronic illness. Southern Online Journal of Nursing Research 2008;8(2):2p. *X-6*

191. Latzman RD, Majumdar S, Bigelow C, et al. Transitioning to adult care among adolescents with sickle cell disease: A transitioning clinic based on patient and caregiver concerns and needs. Int J Child Adolesc Health 2010;3(4):537-45. *X-7*

192. Lawson EF, Hersh AO, Applebaum MA, et al. Self-management skills in adolescents with chronic rheumatic disease: A cross-sectional survey. Pediatr Rheumatol Online J 2011;9(1):35. PMID: 22145642. *X-3*

193. Lawson V. I wasn't the only one. Ment Health Today 2003 Jul-Aug:34-6. PMID: 14625919. *X-3*

194. Lee PJ. Growing older: the adult metabolic clinic. J Inherit Metab Dis 2002 May;25(3):252-60. PMID: 12137234. *X-3*

195. Lefebvre H, Levert MJ. The needs experienced by individuals and their loved ones following a traumatic brain injury. J Trauma Nurs 2012 Oct-Dec;19(4):197-207. PMID: 23222398. *X-1*

196. Lemacks J, Fowles K, Mateus A, et al. Insights from parents about caring for a child with birth defects. Int J Environ Res Public Health. 2013 Aug;10(8):3465-82. PMID: 23965922. *X-6*

197. Leonard BJ, Garwick A, Adwan JZ. Adolescents' perceptions of parental roles and involvement in diabetes management. J Pediatr Nurs 2005 Dec;20(6):405-14. PMID: 16298281. *X-3*

198. Lesch W, Specht K, Lux A, et al. Disease-specific knowledge and information preferences of young patients with congenital heart disease. Cardiol Young 2013 Apr 29:1-10. PMID: 23628281. *X-3*

199. Lewis SA, Noyes J. Effective process or dangerous precipice: qualitative comparative embedded case study with young people with epilepsy and their parents during transition from children's to adult services. BMC Pediatr 2013 Oct 16;13(1):169. PMID: 24131769. *X-5*

200. Lewis SA, Noyes J, Mackereth S. Knowledge and information needs of young people with epilepsy and their parents: Mixed-method systematic review. BMC Pediatr 2010;10:103. PMID: 21194484. *X-3*

201. Libby R. Principles of health care financing. Pediatrics 2010 Nov;126(5):1018-21. PMID: 20974786. *X-2, X-3*

202. Lindgren E, Soderberg S, Skar L. The gap in transition between child and adolescent psychiatry and general adult psychiatry. J Child Adolesc Psychiatr Nurs 2013 May;26(2):103-9. PMID: 23607821. *X-5*

203. Lineham K. Caring for young people with chronic illness: a case study. Paediatr Nurs 2010 Feb;22(1):20-3. PMID: 20302060. *X-4*

204. LoCasale-Crouch J, Johnson B. Transition from pediatric to adult medical care. Adv Chronic Kidney Dis 2005 Oct;12(4):412-7. PMID: 16198281. *X-1*

205. Looman WS, Lindeke LL. Children and youth with special health care needs: partnering with families for effective advocacy. J Pediatr Health Care 2008 Mar-Apr;22(2):134-6. PMID: 18294584. *X-3*

206. Lotstein DS, McPherson M, Strickland B, et al. Transition planning for youth with special health care needs: results from the National Survey of Children with Special Health Care Needs. Pediatrics 2005 Jun;115(6):1562-8. PMID: 15930217. *X-5*

207. Lotstein DS, Seid M, Klingensmith G, et al. Transition from pediatric to adult care for youth diagnosed with type 1 diabetes in adolescence. Pediatrics 2013 Apr;131(4):e1062-70. PMID: 23530167. *X-5*

208. Lubetsky MJ, Handen BL, Lubetsky M, et al. Systems of care for individuals with autism spectrum disorder and serious behavioral disturbance through the lifespan. Child Adolesc Psychiatr Clin N Am 2014 Jan;23(1):97-110. PMID: 24231170. *X-6*

209. Lundin CS, Danielson E, Ohrn I. Handling the transition of adolescents with diabetes: participant observations and interviews with care providers in paediatric and adult diabetes outpatient clinics. Int J Integr Care 2007;7:e05. PMID: 17377641. *X-5*

210. Luyckx K, Goossens E, Van Damme C, et al. Identity formation in adolescents with congenital cardiac disease: a forgotten issue in the transition to

adulthood. Cardiol Young 2011 Aug;21(4):411-20. PMID: 21406136. *X-3, X-4*

211. Lyons SK, Libman IM, Sperling MA. Clinical review: Diabetes in the adolescent: transitional issues. J Clin Endocrinol Metab. 2013 Dec;98(12):4639-45. PMID: 24152689. *X-8*

212. Macdonald S, McLaughlin S, Levey E, et al. One family's journey: Medical Home and the network of supports it offers children and youth with special healthcare needs: the transition process continues. Exceptional Parent 2008;38(5):60-3. *X-6*

213. Macdonald S, Sagerman PJ, Boyd L, et al. One family's journey: Medical Home and the network of supports [sic] it offers children and youth with special healthcare needs: the transition process starts early... part seven. Exceptional Parent 2008;38(4):57-61. *X-6*

214. Majnemer A, Mazer B. New directions in the outcome evaluation of children with cerebral palsy. Semin Pediatr Neurol 2004 Mar;11(1):11-7. PMID: 15132249. *X-3*

215. Mandarino K. Transitional-Age Youths: Barriers to Accessing Adult Mental Health Services and the Changing Definition of Adolescence. Journal of Human Behavior in the Social Environment. 2014;24(4):462-74. PMID: 2012563230. *X-7*

216. Mandelco B, Clark L, Freeborn D, et al. Overview: transition to adulthood: challenges for parents and youth with disabilities. Communicating Nursing Research 2010;43:194-. *X-7*

217. Manzur AY, Muntoni F. Diagnosis and new treatments in muscular dystrophies. J Neurol Neurosurg Psychiatry 2009 Jul;80(7):706-14. PMID: 19531685. *X-6*

218. Manzur AY, Muntoni F. Diagnosis and new treatments in muscular dystrophies. Postgrad Med J 2009 Nov;85(1009):622-30. PMID: 19892898. *X-6*

219. Marcer H, Finlay F, Baverstock A. ADHD and transition to adult services--the experience of community paediatricians. Child Care Health Dev 2008 Sep;34(5):564-6. PMID: 18796048. *X-5*

220. Markowitz JT, Laffel LM. Transitions in care: support group for young adults with Type 1 diabetes. Diabet Med 2012 Apr;29(4):522-5. PMID: 22150392. *X-5*

221. Marshall M, Carter B, Rose K, et al. Living with type 1 diabetes: perceptions of children and their parents. J Clin Nurs 2009 Jun;18(12):1703-10. PMID: 19646116. *X-3*

222. Martin AB, Crawford S, Probst JC, et al. Medical homes for children with special health care needs: a program evaluation. J Health Care Poor Underserved 2007 Nov;18(4):916-30. PMID: 17982215. *X-3*

223. Matlow AG, Wright JG, Zimmerman B, et al. How can the principles of complexity science be applied to improve the coordination of care for complex pediatric patients? Qual Saf Health Care 2006 Apr;15(2):85-8. PMID: 16585105. *X-3*

224. Maunder EZ. The challenge of transitional care for young people with life-limiting illness. Br J Nurs 2004 May 27-Jun 9;13(10):594-6. PMID: 15215714. *X-6*

225. McAllister JW, Presler E, Cooley WC. Practice-based care coordination: a medical home essential. Pediatrics 2007 Sep;120(3):e723-33. PMID: 17766512. *X-3*

226. McClannahan LE, MacDuff GS, Krantz PJ. Behavior analysis and intervention for adults with autism. Behav Modif 2002 Jan;26(1):9-26. PMID: 11799656. *X-4*

227. McCurdy C, DiCenso A, Boblin S, et al. There to here: young adult patients' perceptions of the process of transition from pediatric to adult transplant care. Prog Transplant 2006 Dec;16(4):309-16. PMID: 17183937. *X-5*

228. McDonagh JE. Transition of care from paediatric to adult rheumatology. Arch Dis Child 2007 Sep;92(9):802-7. PMID: 17715444. *X-6*

229. McDonagh JE. Young people first, juvenile idiopathic arthritis second: transitional care in rheumatology. Arthritis Rheum 2008 Aug 15;59(8):1162-70. PMID: 18668608. *X-6*

230. McDonagh JE, Kaufman M. Transition from pediatric to adult care after solid organ transplantation. Curr Opin Organ Transplant 2009 Oct;14(5):526-32. PMID: 19617823. *X-6*

231. McDonagh JE, Kelly DA. Transitioning care of the pediatric recipient to adult caregivers. Pediatr Clin North Am 2003 Dec;50(6):1561-83, xi-xii. PMID: 14710793. *X-6*

232. McGrew JH, Danner M. Evaluation of an intensive case management program for transition age youth and its transition to assertive community treatment. American Journal of Psychiatric Rehabilitation 2009;12(3):278-94. *X-3*

233. McLaughlin S, Bowering N, Crosby B, et al. Health care transition for adolescents with special health care needs: a report on the development and use of a clinical transition service. R I Med J (2013) 2013;96(4):25-7. PMID: 23641448. *X-5*

234. McLaughlin SE, Diener-West M, Indurkhya A, et al. Improving transition from pediatric to adult cystic fibrosis care: lessons from a national survey of current practices. Pediatrics 2008 May;121(5):e1160-6. PMID: 18450860. *X-5*

235. McMillan JA. Growing pains: prepared for transition with nowhere to go. Contemporary Pediatrics 2009;26(12):6-. *X-3*

236. McMillen JC, Raghavan R. Pediatric to adult mental health service use of young people leaving the foster care system. J Adolesc Health 2009 Jan;44(1):7-13. PMID: 19101453. *X-5*

237. McNamara N, McNicholas F, Ford T, et al. Transition from child and adolescent to adult mental health services in the Republic of Ireland: an investigation of process and operational practice. Early Interv Psychiatry 2013 Jul 4PMID: 23826636. *X-5*

238. McPherson M, Thaniel L, Minniti CP. Transition of patients with sickle cell disease from pediatric to adult care: Assessing patient readiness. Pediatr Blood Cancer 2009 Jul;52(7):838-41. PMID: 19229973. *X-5*

239. McPherson M, Weissman G, Strickland BB, et al. Implementing community-based systems of services for children and youths with special health care needs: how well are we doing? Pediatrics 2004 May;113(5 Suppl):1538-44. PMID: 15121923. *X-3*

240. Mennito S. Resident preferences for a curriculum in healthcare transitions for young adults. South Med J 2012 Sep;105(9):462-6. PMID: 22948324. *X-1*

241. Michaud PA, Suris JC, Viner R. The adolescent with a chronic condition. Part II: healthcare provision. Arch Dis Child 2004 Oct;89(10):943-9. PMID: 15383439. *X-3*

242. Milbrath C. Caring for an underserved population: Helping pediatric patients with disabilities transition to adulthood. Creat Nurs 2008;14(2):66-9. PMID: 18655515. *X-6*

243. Miles K, Edwards S, Clapson M. Transition from paediatric to adult services: experiences of HIV-positive adolescents. AIDS Care 2004 Apr;16(3):305-14. PMID: 15203424. *X-5*

244. Miller D, MacDonald D. Management of pediatric patients with chronic kidney disease. Pediatr Nurs 2006 Mar-Apr;32(2):128-34; quiz 35. PMID: 16719422. *X-3*

245. Miller VA, Harris D. Measuring children's decision-making involvement regarding chronic illness management. J Pediatr Psychol 2012 Apr;37(3):292-306. PMID: 22138318. *X-3*

246. Mills J, Cutajar P, Jones J, et al. Ensuring the successful transition of adolescents to adult services. Learning Disability Practice 2013;16(6):26-8. *X-5*

247. Moons P, De Geest S, Budts W. Comprehensive care for adults with congenital heart disease: expanding roles for nurses. Eur J Cardiovasc Nurs 2002 Feb;1(1):23-8. PMID: 14622863. *X-6*

248. Moorthy LN, Peterson MG, Hassett AL, et al. Burden of childhood-onset arthritis. Pediatr Rheumatol Online J 2010;8:20. PMID: 20615240. *X-6*

249. Munson MR, Jaccard J, Smalling SE, et al. Static, dynamic, integrated, and contextualized: a framework for understanding mental health service utilization among young adults. Soc Sci Med 2012 Oct;75(8):1441-9. PMID: 22800921. *X-3*

250. Musallam K, Cappellini MD, Taher A. Challenges associated with prolonged survival of patients with thalassemia: transitioning from childhood to adulthood. Pediatrics 2008 May;121(5):e1426-9. PMID: 18450884. *X-6*

251. Mutze U, Roth A, Weigel JF, et al. Transition of young adults with phenylketonuria from pediatric to adult care. J Inherit Metab Dis 2011 Jun;34(3):701-9. PMID: 21305352. *X-5*

252. Myers CT. Exploring occupational therapy and transitions for young children with special needs.

Phys Occup Ther Pediatr 2006;26(3):73-88. PMID: 16966317. *X-3*

253. Nakhla M, Daneman D, Frank M, et al. Translating transition: a critical review of the diabetes literature. J Pediatr Endocrinol Metab 2008 Jun;21(6):507-16. PMID: 18717235. *X-6*

254. Neff JM, Clifton H, Park KJ, et al. Identifying children with lifelong chronic conditions for care coordination by using hospital discharge data. Acad Pediatr 2010 Nov-Dec;10(6):417-23. PMID: 21075324. *X-3*

255. Neu A, Losch-Binder M, Ehehalt S, et al. Follow-up of adolescents with diabetes after transition from paediatric to adult care: results of a 10-year prospective study. Exp Clin Endocrinol Diabetes 2010 Jun;118(6):353-5. PMID: 20140851. *X-5*

256. Nutt DJ, Fone K, Asherson P, et al. Evidence-based guidelines for management of attention-deficit/hyperactivity disorder in adolescents in transition to adult services and in adults: recommendations from the British Association for Psychopharmacology. J Psychopharmacol 2007 Jan;21(1):10-41. PMID: 17092962. *X-6*

257. O'Connor KS, Brooks KS, Nysse-Carris KL, et al. Design and operation of the Survey of Adult Transition and Health, 2007. Vital Health Stat 1 2011 Mar(52):1-85. PMID: 21548442. *X-1*

258. Oftedahl E, Benedict R, Katcher ML. National survey of children with special health care needs: Wisconsin-specific data. WMJ 2004;103(5):88-90. PMID: 15553573. *X-3*

259. Okumura MJ, Heisler M, Davis MM, et al. Comfort of general internists and general pediatricians in providing care for young adults with chronic illnesses of childhood. J Gen Intern Med 2008 Oct;23(10):1621-7. PMID: 18661191. *X-5*

260. Onyeajam DJ, Eke R, Stephens TG, et al. Time to linkage to care and viro-immunologic parameters of individuals diagnosed before and after the 2006 HIV testing recommendations. South Med J 2013 Apr;106(4):257-66. PMID: 23558414. *X-1, X-3*

261. Oskoui M. Growing up with cerebral palsy: contemporary challenges of healthcare transition. Can J Neurol Sci 2012 Jan;39(1):23-5. PMID: 22384484. *X-6*

262. Ostlie IL, Dale O, Moller A. From childhood to adult life with juvenile idiopathic arthritis (JIA): a pilot study. Disabil Rehabil 2007 Mar 30;29(6):445-52. PMID: 17364799. *X-5*

263. Oswald DP, Bodurtha JN, Willis JH, et al. Underinsurance and key health outcomes for children with special health care needs. Pediatrics 2007 Feb;119(2):e341-7. PMID: 17210727. *X-5*

264. Owen P, Beskine D. Factors affecting transition of young people with diabetes. Paediatr Nurs 2008 Sep;20(7):33-8. PMID: 18808056. *X-6*

265. Pacaud D. Editorial commentary. Bridge over troubled water: improving the transition from pediatric to adult care. The pediatric care perspective. Canadian Journal of Diabetes 2005;29(3):183-4. *X-6*

266. Pacaud D, Yale J, Stephure D, et al. Problems in transition from pediatric care to adult care for individuals with diabetes. Canadian Journal of Diabetes 2005;29(1):13-8. *X-5*

267. Pacaud D, Yale JF. Exploring a black hole: Transition from paediatric to adult care services for youth with diabetes. Paediatr Child Health 2005 Jan;10(1):31-4. PMID: 19657443. *X-6*

268. Pakdeeprom B, In-Iw S, Chintanadilok N, et al. Promoting factors for transition readiness of adolescent chronic illnesses: experiences in Thailand. J Med Assoc Thai 2012 Aug;95(8):1028-34. PMID: 23061306. *X-5*

269. Palmer J, Glah C, Zelikovsky N, et al. A Collaborative Approach to the Transition of Adolescent Renal Transplant Recipients to Adult Care Providers. Nephrology Nursing Journal 2011;38(2):200-. *X-5*

270. Papagianni M, Stanhope R. How should we manage growth hormone deficiency in adolescence? Transition from paediatric to adult care. J Pediatr Endocrinol Metab 2003 Jan;16(1):23-5. PMID: 12585336. *X-6*

271. Parachuri V, Inglese C. Neurological problems in the adolescent population. Adolesc Med State Art Rev 2013 Apr;24(1):1-28. PMID: 23705516. *X-3, X-6*

272. Parfitt G. Imroving young person's experience transition: lessons from Wales. Paediatr Nurs 2008 Nov;20(9):27-30. PMID: 19006948. *X-6*

D-14

273. Parr C. Ensuring equity in diabetes care. Independent Nurse 2012:10-. *X-3*

274. Patterson D. Promoting successful transition from pediatric to adult-oriented health care. Exceptional Parent 2004;34(3):56. *X-6*

275. Paul M, Ford T, Kramer T, et al. Transfers and transitions between child and adult mental health services. Br J Psychiatry Suppl 2013 Jan;54:s36-40. PMID: 23288500. *X-5*

276. Pearson GS, Hawke JM, Dundon E, et al. Timely help for troubled youth. Behav Healthc 2010 Mar;30(3):31-3. PMID: 20373689. *X-3*

277. Pedreira CC, Hameed R, Kanumakala S, et al. Health-care problems of Turner syndrome in the adult woman: a cross sectional study of a Victorian cohort and a case for transition. Intern Med J 2006 Jan;36(1):54-7. PMID: 16409314. *X-1, X-3*

278. Perry L, Lowe JM, Steinbeck KS, et al. Services doing the best they can: service experiences of young adults with type 1 diabetes mellitus in rural Australia. J Clin Nurs 2012 Jul;21(13-14):1955-63. PMID: 22672458. *X-5*

279. Petitgout JM, Pelzer DE, McConkey SA, et al. Development of a hospital-based care coordination program for children with special health care needs. J Pediatr Health Care. 2013 Nov-Dec;27(6):419-25. PMID: 22575784. *X-5*

280. Philpott JR. Transitional care in inflammatory bowel disease. Gastroenterol Hepatol (N Y) 2011 Jan;7(1):26-32. PMID: 21346849. *X-6*

281. Pickler L, Kellar-Guenther Y, Goldson E. Barriers to transition to adult care for youth with intellectual disabilities. International Journal of Child and Adolescent Health 2010 2012-09-10;3(4):575-84. *X-7*

282. Pilnick A, Clegg J, Murphy E, et al. Questioning the answer: questioning style, choice and self-determination in interactions with young people with intellectual disabilities. Sociol Health Illn 2010 Mar;32(3):415-36. PMID: 20415789. *X-4*

283. Porter JS, Graff JC, Lopez AD, et al. Transition From Pediatric to Adult Care in Sickle Cell Disease: Perspectives on the Family Role. J Pediatr Nurs 2013 Oct 16PMID: 24188784. *X-5*

284. Price C, Corbett S, Dovey-Pearce G. Barriers and facilitators to implementing a transition pathway for adolescents with diabetes: A health professionals perspective. International Journal of Child and Adolescent Health 2010 2012-09-10;3(4):489-98. *X-7*

285. Price CS, Corbett S, Lewis-Barned N, et al. Implementing a transition pathway in diabetes: a qualitative study of the experiences and suggestions of young people with diabetes. Child Care Health Dev 2011 Nov;37(6):852-60. PMID: 22007985. *X-5*

286. Punch R, Hyde M, Creed PA. Issues in the school-to-work transition of hard of hearing adolescents. Am Ann Deaf 2004 Spring;149(1):28-38. PMID: 15332464. *X-3, X-4*

287. Punpanich W, Detels R, Gorbach PM, et al. Understanding the psychosocial needs of HIV-infected children and families: a qualitative study. J Med Assoc Thai 2008 Oct;91 Suppl 3:S76-84. PMID: 19253500. *X-3*

288. Quinn CT, Rogers ZR, McCavit TL, et al. Improved survival of children and adolescents with sickle cell disease. Blood 2010 Apr 29;115(17):3447-52. PMID: 20194891. *X-3*

289. Rasmussen B, Wellard S, Nankervis A. Consumer issues in navigating health care services for type I diabetes. J Clin Nurs 2001 Sep;10(5):628-34. PMID: 11822513. *X-5*

290. Read N, Schofield A. Autism: are mental health services failing children and parents? J Fam Health Care 2010;20(4):120-4. PMID: 21053660. *X-3*

291. Reading R. Lost in transition? Between paediatric and adult services. Child: Care, Health & Development 2006;32(4):501-2. *X-6*

292. Rekate HL. The pediatric neurosurgical patient: the challenge of growing up. Semin Pediatr Neurol 2009 Mar;16(1):2-8. PMID: 19410150. *X-6*

293. Remorino R, Taylor J. Smoothing things over: the transition from pediatric to adult care for kidney transplant recipients. Prog Transplant 2006 Dec;16(4):303-8. PMID: 17183936. *X-5*

294. Rideout K. Evaluation of a PNP care coordinator model for hospitalized children, adolescents, and young adults with cystic fibrosis. Pediatr Nurs 2007 Jan-Feb;33(1):29-35; quiz -6. PMID: 17410998. *X-3*

295. Ritholz MD, Wolpert H, Beste M, et al. Patient-Provider Relationships Across the Transition From Pediatric to Adult Diabetes Care: A Qualitative Study. Diabetes Educ 2013 Nov 20PMID: 24258251. *X-5*

296. Robertson LP, McDonagh JE, Southwood TR, et al. Growing up and moving on. A multicentre UK audit of the transfer of adolescents with juvenile idiopathic arthritis from paediatric to adult centred care. Ann Rheum Dis 2006 Jan;65(1):74-80. PMID: 15994281. *X-5*

297. Rook M, Rosenthal P. Caring for adults with pediatric liver disease. Curr Gastroenterol Rep 2009 Feb;11(1):83-9. PMID: 19166664. *x-6*

298. Rosenberg D, Onufer C, Clark G, et al. The need for care coordination among children with special health care needs in Illinois. Matern Child Health J 2005 Jun;9(2 Suppl):S41-7. PMID: 15973478. *X-3*

299. Ross AC, Camacho-Gonzalez A, Henderson S, et al. The HIV-Infected Adolescent. Curr Infect Dis Rep 2010 Jan;12(1):63-70. PMID: 21308499. *X-6*

300. Rouse CM. Informing choice or teaching submission to medical authority: a case study of adolescent transitioning for sickle cell patients. Ethn Health 2011 Aug-Oct;16(4-5):313-25. PMID: 21797720. *X-3*

301. Rubin K. Transitioning the patient with Turner's syndrome from pediatric to adult care. J Pediatr Endocrinol Metab 2003 May;16 Suppl 3:651-9. PMID: 12795368. *X-7*

302. Rubin KR. Turner syndrome: transition from pediatrics to adulthood. Endocr Pract 2008 Sep;14(6):775-81. PMID: 18996801. *X-6*

303. Ruck J, Dahan-Oliel N. Adolescence and young adulthood in spina bifida: self-report on care received and readiness for the future. Topics in Spinal Cord Injury Rehabilitation 2010;16(1):26-37. *X-5*

304. Rudy C. When do pediatric patients graduate? J Pediatr Health Care 2006 Sep-Oct;20(5):334-5, 58-60. PMID: 16962439. *X-6*

305. Saidi A, Reiss J, Breitinger P, et al. Web-based learning: Is it an effective method for educating pediatric residents about transition to adult subspecialty congenital heart disease care?

International Journal of Child and Adolescent Health 2010 2012-09-10;3(4):585-93. *X-7*

306. Sakakibara H, Yoshida H, Takei M, et al. Health management of adults with Turner syndrome: an attempt at multidisciplinary medical care by gynecologists in cooperation with specialists from other fields. J Obstet Gynaecol Res 2011 Jul;37(7):836-42. PMID: 21410832. *X-1*

307. Samyn M. Optimizing outcomes for pediatric recipients. Liver Transpl 2012 Nov;18 Suppl 2:S34-8. PMID: 22941584. *X-6*

308. Scal P, Davern M, Ireland M, et al. Transition to adulthood: delays and unmet needs among adolescents and young adults with asthma. J Pediatr 2008 Apr;152(4):471-5, 5 e1. PMID: 18346498. *X-3*

309. Scal P, Garwick A, Horvath KJ. Making Rheumtogrow: The rationale and framework for an Internet based health care transition intervention. International Journal of Child and Adolescent Health 2010 2012-09-10;3(4):451-61. *X-7*

310. Scal P, Horvath K, Garwick A. Preparing for adulthood: health care transition counseling for youth with arthritis. Arthritis Rheum 2009 Jan 15;61(1):52-7. PMID: 19116976. *X-5*

311. Scal P, Ireland M. Addressing transition to adult health care for adolescents with special health care needs. Pediatrics 2005 Jun;115(6):1607-12. PMID: 15930223. *X-5*

312. Schor NF. Life at the interface: Adults with "pediatric" disorders of the nervous system. Ann Neurol 2013 Apr 11PMID: 23575604. *X-6*

313. Schrans DG, Abbott D, Peay HL, et al. Transition in Duchenne muscular dystrophy: An expert meeting report and description of transition needs in an emergent patient population: (Parent Project Muscular Dystrophy Transition Expert Meeting 17-18 June 2011, Amsterdam, The Netherlands). Neuromuscul Disord 2013 Mar;23(3):283-6. PMID: 22989602. *X-6*

314. Schultz RJ. Parental experiences of transitioning their adolescent with epilepsy and cognitive impairments from pediatric to adult health care: Texas Woman's University; 2009.

315. Schultz RJ. Parental experiences transitioning their adolescent with epilepsy and cognitive impairments to adult health care. J Pediatr Health

Care 2013 Sep-Oct;27(5):359-66. PMID: 22560804. *X-5*

316. Schwartz LA, Brumley LD, Tuchman LK, et al. Stakeholder validation of a model of readiness for transition to adult care. JAMA Pediatr 2013 Oct;167(10):939-46. PMID: 23959392. *X-2*

317. Scott LK. Developmental mastery of diabetes-related tasks in children. Nurs Clin North Am 2013 Jun;48(2):329-42. PMID: 23659817. *X-3, X-6*

318. Serra MF, McCarthy C. Pediatric rehabilitation day treatment for children with brain injury and neurodevelopmental disorders. Med Health R I 2010 Apr;93(4):103-5. PMID: 20486519. *X-4*

319. Shapiro JR, Germain-Lee EL. Osteogenesis imperfecta: effecting the transition from adolescent to adult medical care. J Musculoskelet Neuronal Interact 2012 Mar;12(1):24-7. PMID: 22373948. *X-6*

320. Sharma N, Willen E, Garcia A, et al. Attitudes Toward Transitioning in Youth With Perinatally Acquired HIV and Their Family Caregivers. J Assoc Nurses AIDS Care 2013 Jun 25 PMID: 23809660. *X-5*

321. Sharma N, Willen E, Garcia A, et al. Attitudes toward transitioning in youth with perinatally acquired HIV and their family caregivers. J Assoc Nurses AIDS Care 2014 Mar-Apr;25(2):168-75. PMID: 23809660. *X-8*

322. Shaw KL, Southwood TR, McDonagh JE. Growing up and moving on in rheumatology: a multicentre cohort of adolescents with juvenile idiopathic arthritis. Rheumatology (Oxford) 2005 Jun;44(6):806-12. PMID: 15769786. *X-5*

323. Shaw KL, Southwood TR, McDonagh JE. Development and preliminary validation of the 'Mind the Gap' scale to assess satisfaction with transitional health care among adolescents with juvenile idiopathic arthritis. Child Care Health Dev 2007 Jul;33(4):380-8. PMID: 17584392. *X-5*

324. Shulman ST. Complex care is complicated! Pediatr Ann 2010 Apr;39(4):183-4. PMID: 20411892. *X-3*

325. Simmonds J, Burch M. Shared care in paediatric heart transplantation. Arch Dis Child Educ Pract Ed 2008 Apr;93(2):37-43. PMID: 18356304. *X-3*

326. Singh SP. Transition of care from child to adult mental health services: the great divide. Curr Opin Psychiatry 2009 Jul;22(4):386-90. PMID: 19417667. *X-6*

327. Singh SP, Paul M, Ford T, et al. Process, outcome and experience of transition from child to adult mental healthcare: multiperspective study. Br J Psychiatry 2010 Oct;197(4):305-12. PMID: 20884954. *X-5*

328. Smith K. Asthma management in children. Nebr Nurse 2004 Jun-Aug;37(2):26-8; quiz 8-9. PMID: 15233013. *X-3*

329. Sneed RC, May WL, Stencel C. Policy versus practice: comparison of prescribing therapy and durable medical equipment in medical and educational settings. Pediatrics 2004 Nov;114(5):e612-25. PMID: 15520092. *X-3*

330. Sommelet D. Chronic pediatric diseases into adulthood and the challenge of adolescence. Handb Clin Neurol. 2013;111:101-5. PMID: 23622155. *X-6*

331. Spaic T, Mahon JL, Hramiak I, et al. Multicentre randomized controlled trial of structured transition on diabetes care management compared to standard diabetes care in adolescents and young adults with type 1 diabetes (Transition Trial). BMC Pediatr 2013;13:163. PMID: 24106787. *X-6*

332. Spears AP. The Healthy People 2010 outcomes for the care of children with special health care needs: an effective national policy for meeting mental health care needs? Matern Child Health J 2010 May;14(3):401-11. PMID: 18256914. *X-3*

333. Speiser PW. Congenital adrenal hyperplasia: transition from chil dhood to adulthood. J Endocrinol Invest 2001 Oct;24(9):681-91. PMID: 11716155. *X-3*

334. Spiegel HM, Futterman DC. Adolescents and HIV: prevention and clinical care. Curr HIV/AIDS Rep 2009 May;6(2):100-7. PMID: 19358781. *X-6*

335. Steinbeck K, Brodie L. Bringing in the voices: a transition forum for young people with chronic illness or disability. Neonatal, Paediatric & Child Health Nursing 2006;9(1):22-6. *X-6*

336. Stein M. Young People's Transitions from Care to Adulthood in European and Postcommunist Eastern European and Central Asian Societies. Australian Social Work. 2014;67(1):24-38. PMID: 2012506653. *X-7*

337. Steinkamp G, Ullrich G, Muller C, et al. Transition of adult patients with cystic fibrosis from paediatric to adult care--the patients' perspective before and after start-up of an adult clinic. Eur J Med Res 2001 Feb 28;6(2):85-92. PMID: 11313196. *X-1*

338. Sterling L, Nyhof-Young J, Blanchette VS, et al. Exploring internet needs and use among adolescents with haemophilia: a website development project. Haemophilia 2012 Mar;18(2):216-21. PMID: 21797947. *X-3, X-4*

339. Stewart D, Stavness C, King G, et al. A critical appraisal of literature reviews about the transition to adulthood for youth with disabilities. Phys Occup Ther Pediatr 2006;26(4):5-24. PMID: 17135067. *X-4*

340. Sullivan WF, Berg JM, Bradley E, et al. Primary care of adults with developmental disabilities: Canadian consensus guidelines. Can Fam Physician 2011 May;57(5):541-53, e154-68. PMID: 21571716. *X-6*

341. Swift KD, Hall CL, Marimuttu V, et al. Transition to adult mental health services for young people with attention deficit/hyperactivity disorder (ADHD): a qualitative analysis of their experiences. BMC Psychiatry 2013;13:74. PMID: 23497082. *X-5*

342. Taylor A, Lizzi M, Marx A, et al. Implementing a care coordination program for children with special healthcare needs: partnering with families and providers. J Healthc Qual 2013 Sep;35(5):70-7. PMID: 22913270. *X-3*

343. Taylor L, Tsang A, Drabble A. Transition of transplant patients with cystic fibrosis to adult care: today's challenges. Prog Transplant 2006 Dec;16(4):329-34; quiz 35. PMID: 17183940. *X-6*

344. Thrall RS, Blumberg JH, Beck S, et al. Beyond the medical home: Special Care Family Academy for children and youth. Pediatr Nurs 2012 Nov-Dec;38(6):331-5. PMID: 23362633. *X-6*

345. Thurgate C. Living with disability: Part 3. Communication and care. Paediatr Nurs 2006 Jun;18(5):40-4. PMID: 16784064. *X-3*

346. Tong A, Wong G, Hodson E, et al. Adolescent views on transition in diabetes and nephrology. Eur J Pediatr 2013 Mar;172(3):293-304. PMID: 22576804. *X-5*

347. Tracy J, Henderson D. Children and adolescents with developmental disabilities. The GP's role. Aust Fam Physician 2004 Aug;33(8):591-7. PMID: 15373375. *X-3*

348. Tsamasiros J, Bartsocas CS. Transition of the adolescent from the children's to the adults' diabetes clinic. J Pediatr Endocrinol Metab 2002 Apr;15(4):363-7. PMID: 12008681. *X-6*

349. Tuchman L, Schwartz M. Health outcomes associated with transition from pediatric to adult cystic fibrosis care. Pediatrics 2013 Nov;132(5):847-53. PMID: 24144711. *X-3, X-5*

350. Tuchman LK, Slap GB, Britto MT. Transition to adult care: experiences and expectations of adolescents with a chronic illness. Child Care Health Dev 2008 Sep;34(5):557-63. PMID: 18796047. *X-5*

351. Valcarcel T. Role of the primary care provider in transitioning patients with juvenile arthritis. Pediatr Ann. 2012 Nov;41(11):469-70. PMID: 23814935. *X-6*

352. Valenzuela JM, Buchanan CL, Radcliffe J, et al. Transition to adult services among behaviorally infected adolescents with HIV--a qualitative study. J Pediatr Psychol 2011 Mar;36(2):134-40. PMID: 19542198. *X-5*

353. van den Heuvel ME, van der Lee JH, Cornelissen EA, et al. Transition to the adult nephrologist does not induce acute renal transplant rejection. Nephrol Dial Transplant 2010 May;25(5):1662-7. PMID: 20026560. *X-5*

354. van der Toorn M, Cobussen-Boekhorst H, Kwak K, et al. Needs of children with a chronic bladder in preparation for transfer to adult care. J Pediatr Urol. 2013 Aug;9(4):509-15. PMID: 22695375. *X-5*

355. van Pelt PA, Kruize AA, Goren SS, et al. Transition of rheumatologic care, from teenager to adult: which health assessment questionnaire can be best used? Clin Exp Rheumatol 2010 Mar-Apr;28(2):281-6. PMID: 20483054. *X-3*

356. Van Riper CL, Wallace LS. Position of the American Dietetic Association: Providing nutrition services for people with developmental disabilities and special health care needs. J Am Diet Assoc 2010 Feb;110(2):296-307. PMID: 20112461. *X-6*

357. van Staa A, van der Stege HA, Jedeloo S, et al. Readiness to transfer to adult care of adolescents with chronic conditions: exploration of associated factors.

J Adolesc Health 2011 Mar;48(3):295-302. PMID: 21338902. *X-5*

358. Van Walleghem N. Editorial commentary. Bridging the gap: transition from pediatric to adult diabetes care. Canadian Journal of Diabetes 2005;29(1):10-1. *X-6*

359. Vinchon M, Dhellemmes P. The transition from child to adult in neurosurgery. Adv Tech Stand Neurosurg 2007;32:3-24. PMID: 17907472. *X-5*

360. Visentin K, Koch T, Kralik D. Adolescents with Type 1 Diabetes: transition between diabetes services. J Clin Nurs 2006 Jun;15(6):761-9. PMID: 16684172. *X-5*

361. Volta C, Luppino T, Street ME, et al. Transition from pediatric to adult care of children with chronic endocrine diseases: a survey on the current modalities in Italy. J Endocrinol Invest 2003 Feb;26(2):157-62. PMID: 12739744. *X-5*

362. Waite A. Helping Adolescents With CP Transition Into Adulthood. OT Practice. 2014;19(3):5-. PMID: 2012488707. *X-6*

363. Waite E, Laraque D. Pediatric organ transplant patients and long-term care: a review. Mt Sinai J Med 2006 Dec;73(8):1148-55. PMID: 17285215. *X-6*

364. Wan J. Adolescent urology update. Adolesc Med State Art Rev 2013 Apr;24(1):273-94. PMID: 23705530. *X-2, X-3, X-4, X-6*

365. Warren-Boulton E, Gallivan JM. Pediatric to Adult Care Transition Challenges and NDEP Resources... National Diabetes Education Program. School Nurse News 2011;28(3):29-31. *X-3*

366. Watson AR, Shooter M. Transitioning adolescents from pediatric to adult dialysis units. Adv Perit Dial 1996;12:176-8. PMID: 8865896. *X-6*

367. Watson L. Too old at 18: a parent's view of transition. Paediatr Nurs 2006 Sep;18(7):25. PMID: 16986752. *X-6*

368. Webb AK, Jones AW, Dodd ME. Transition from paediatric to adult care: problems that arise in the adult cystic fibrosis clinic. J R Soc Med 2001;94 Suppl 40:8-11. PMID: 11601165. *X-6*

369. Wells CK, McMorris BJ, Horvath KJ, et al. Youth report of healthcare transition counseling and autonomy support from their rheumatologist. Pediatr Rheumatol Online J 2012;10(1):36. PMID: 23151125. *X-5*

370. While AE, Mullen J. Living with sickle cell disease: the perspective of young people. Br J Nurs 2004 Mar 25-Apr 7;13(6):320-5. PMID: 15126965. *X-4*

371. White PH. Transition: a future promise for children and adolescents with special health care needs and disabilities. Rheum Dis Clin North Am 2002 Aug;28(3):687-703, viii. PMID: 12380376. *X-6*

372. Wiener LS, Zobel M, Battles H, et al. Transition from a pediatric HIV intramural clinical research program to adolescent and adult community-based care services: assessing transition readiness. Soc Work Health Care 2007;46(1):1-19. PMID: 18032153. *X-1, X-3*

373. Wilens TE, Rosenbaum JF. Transitional aged youth: a new frontier in child and adolescent psychiatry. J Am Acad Child Adolesc Psychiatry. 2013 Sep;52(9):887-90. PMID: 23972688. *X-6*

374. Williams WG. Advanced practice nurses in a medical home. J Spec Pediatr Nurs 2006 Jul;11(3):203-6. PMID: 16774532. *X-3*

375. Wills KE, Nelson SC, Hennessy J, et al. Transition planning for youth with sickle cell disease: embedding neuropsychological assessment into comprehensive care. Pediatrics 2010 Dec;126 Suppl 3:S151-9. PMID: 21123479. *X-3*

376. Witchel SF, Recabarren SE, Gonzalez F, et al. Emerging concepts about prenatal genesis, aberrant metabolism and treatment paradigms in polycystic ovary syndrome. Endocrine 2012 Dec;42(3):526-34. PMID: 22661293. *X-3*

377. Withers AL. Management issues for adolescents with cystic fibrosis. Pulm Med 2012;2012:134132. PMID: 22991662. *X-6*

378. Wolfstadt J, Kaufman A, Levitin J, et al. The use and usefulness of My Health Passport: An online tool for the creation of a portable health summary. International Journal of Child and Adolescent Health 2010 2012-09-10;3(4):499-506. *X-5*

379. Wong LH, Chan FW, Wong FY, et al. Transition care for adolescents and families with chronic illnesses. J Adolesc Health 2010 Dec;47(6):540-6. PMID: 21094430. *X-5*

380. Wood D, Reiss JG, Ferris ME, et al. Transition from pediatric to adult care. International Journal of Child and Adolescent Health 2010 2012-09-10;3(4):445-7. *X-3*

381. Wood E. The child with cerebral palsy: diagnosis and beyond. Semin Pediatr Neurol 2006 Dec;13(4):286-96. PMID: 17178359. *X-6*

382. Wren C, O'Sullivan JJ. Survival with congenital heart disease and need for follow up in adult life. Heart 2001 Apr;85(4):438-43. PMID: 11250973. *X-5*

383. Wynn K, Stewart D, Law M, et al. Creating connections: a community capacity-building project with parents and youth with disabilities in transition to adulthood. Phys Occup Ther Pediatr 2006;26(4):89-103. PMID: 17135071. *X-4*

384. Young G. From boy to man: recommendations for the transition process in haemophilia. Haemophilia 2012 Jul;18 Suppl 5:27-32. PMID: 22757681. *X-3*

385. Zabel TA, Linroth R, Fairman AD. The Life Course Model Web site: an online transition-focused resource for the spina bifida community. Pediatr Clin North Am 2010 Aug;57(4):911-7. PMID: 20883881. *X-3, X-4*

386. Zebracki K, Anderson CJ, Chlan KM, et al. Outcomes of adults with pediatric-onset spinal cord injury: longitudinal findings and implications on transition to adulthood. Topics in Spinal Cord Injury Rehabilitation 2010;16(1):17-25. *X-6*

Appendix E. Ongoing Studies

Study Name Location Trial Identifier	Sponsors and Collaborators Study Status	Population Disease/Condition Age	Interventions / Groups	Primary Outcome Measures
Transition of Adolescents and Young Adults with Diabetes from Pediatric to Adult Care University of Kansas Medical Center Research Institute NCT01109797	Kurt Midyett, MD, CDE Completed, results not published Start: April 2010 Complete: May 2012	• Type I Diabetes or type 2 diabetes managed with insulin • Age 16-29	**Behavioral**: Transition Social Behavioral Intervention **Behavioral**: Diabetes Transition Clinic	• change in self-efficacy • change in diabetes knowledge diabetes quality of life • family conflict • treatment satisfaction
Diabetes Care Management Compared to Standard Diabetes Care in Adolescents and Young Adults with Type 1 Diabetes (TransClin) University of Western Ontario, Canada NCT01351857	University of Western Ontario, Canada Juvenile Diabetes Research Foundation Recruiting Start: April 2012 Complete: December 2016	• T1D diagnosis • Age 17-20	**Other**: Transition Coordinator	• change in one outpatient adult endocrinology visit
Primary Care Transition Study Children's Hospital of Philadelphia NCT01750892	Children's Hospital of Philadelphia Enrolling by invitation Start: October 2012 Complete: December 2013	• 1 chronic condition and/or cognitive disability • Age 19 or older	**Behavioral**: REACH for Independence **Behavioral**: Transition Consult **Other**: Study Materials	• Successful transition to an adult provider
Adolescent, Caregiver, and Young Adult Perspectives of the Transition from Pediatric to Adult Care for Sickle Cell Disease: A Preliminary Evaluation of the Sickle Cell Disease Transition Program St. Jude Children's Research Hospital NCT01569971	St. Jude Children's Research Hospital Plough Foundation Health Resources and Services Administration Recruiting Start: March 2012 Complete: September 2013	• Adolescents with SCD • Young Adults with SCD • Age 12-30	**Other**: Assessment (focus groups and questionnaires)	• Grounded theory qualitative analysis of data

Study Name Location Trial Identifier	Sponsors and Collaborators Study Status	Population Disease/Condition Age	Interventions / Groups	Primary Outcome Measures
The LETS Study: A Longitudinal Evaluation of Transition Services Holland Bloorview Kids Rehabilitation Hospital, Toronto, Ontario, Canada NCT00975338	Holland Bloorview Kids Rehabilitation Hospital Neurotrauma Foundation Active, not recruiting Start: September 2009 Complete: September 2013	• Diagnosis of cerebral palsy or acquired brain injury • Diagnosis of spina bifida • Age 16-23	**Other:** Prospective LIFEspan **Other:** Prospective Non-LIFEspan **Other:** Retrospective Non-LIFEspan	• Maintenance of continuous care
Congenital Heart Adolescents: Program of Transition Evaluation Research (CHAPTER) University of Alberta NCT01286480	Not reported Active, not recruiting Start: January 2011 Complete: December 2012	• Moderate or complex congenital heart disease or acquired heart disease • Age 15-17	**Behavioral:** Clinic-based Educational Intervention	• change in patient satisfaction questionnaire (PSQ-18) • change in parent/guardian Patient Satisfaction Questionnaire (PSQ-18) • change in patient knowledge of his/her CHD (MyHeart score)
The CHAPTER II Study-Congenital Heart Adolescents Participating in Transition Evaluation Research University of Alberta NCT01723332	University of Alberta Heart and Stroke Foundation of Canada Recruiting Start: November 2012 Complete: May 2015	• Moderate or complex CHD • Age 16-17	**Behavioral:** Educational **Behavioral:** Self-management	• Excess time to first ACHD clinic appointment
Transition Study of Inflammatory Bowel Disease (IBD) Patients from Pediatric Gastroenterologist to Adult Gastroenterologist Vanderbilt University NCT00360022	Vanderbilt University Unknown Start: August 2006 Complete: December 2012	• Confirmed diagnosis of IBD • Age 16 and older	**Other:** Transition program	• Decrease IBD flare at 1 year
Implementation of a Pediatric-to-Adult Asthma Transition Program University of Calgary NCT01521247	University of Calgary Recruiting Start: April 2010 Complete: December 2013	• Clinical diagnosis of asthma • Age 17-19	**Other:** Asthma Transition Program	• Asthma Quality of Life Questionnaire with Standardized Activities

Study Name Location Trial Identifier	Sponsors and Collaborators Study Status	Population Disease/Condition Age	Interventions / Groups	Primary Outcome Measures
Internet-based Educational Program to Promote Self-Management for Teens with Hemophilia The Hospital for Sick Children NCT01477437	The Hospital for Sick Children, Toronto, Canada Completed Start: November 2011 Complete: March 2013	• Diagnosis of mild, moderate or severe hemophilia A or B • Age 13-18	**Other:** Teens Taking Charge: Managing Hemophilia Online-Online self-management intervention	• Disease-specific knowledge gained
Long-term Survival with HIV: Psychological and Behavioral Factors Associated with the Transition from Adolescence to Young Adulthood National Cancer Institute NCT00026806	National Cancer Institute Completed Start: July 2001 Complete: June 2005	• HIV-infected adolescents • Age 13-24	NA	• NA
Health literacy-disparities and transition in teens with special healthcare needs Research Institute Nationwide Children's Hospital Medicaid managed plan in Southwest Ohio 5R01MD007160-03	National Institutes of Health National Institute on Minority Health and Health Disparities Ongoing Start: September 2011 End: July 2016	• Special healthcare need • Age 15-17	NA	• NA
Outcomes after transfer of pediatric renal transplant patients to adult providers University of Virginia 5F31NR011237-02	National Institute of Nursing Research Completed Start: August 2009 End: May 2011	• Kidney transplant recipients • Ages 16-25	NA	• NA
From adolescence to adulthood: persons with and without diabetes Carnegie-Mellon University 5R01DK060586-12	National Institutes of Health National Institute of Diabetes and Digestive and Kidney Diseases Ongoing Start: July 2013 End: June 2017	• Diabetes • Ages 22-24	NA	• NA

Study Name Location Trial Identifier	Sponsors and Collaborators Study Status	Population Disease/Condition Age	Interventions / Groups	Primary Outcome Measures
Transitioning from childhood to adulthood: the impact of perinatal HIV infection New York State Psychiatric Institute 5R01MH069133-10	National Institute of Mental Health Ongoing Start: December 2012 End: November 2013	• Perinatally HIV infected youth • Perinatally HIV exposed, uninfected youth	NA	• NA
Barriers & facilitators to health care: transitioning youth with special needs Okumura, Megie University of California, San Francisco AHRQ 5K08HS017716-05 HSRP20084171	Agency for Healthcare Research and Quality Ongoing Start: September 2012 End: September 2013	• Youth and young adults complex chronic conditions	NA	• NA
Cystic fibrosis as a model of health care transition for chronically ill youth Children's Hospital Corporation 5K23HL105541-03	National Heart, Lung, and Blood Institute Ongoing Start: July 2012 End: June 2016	• Adolescents and young adults with cystic fibrosis	NA	• NA
Patient-provider interventions to improve transition to adult care in SCD Cincinnati Children's Hospital Medical Center 5K07HL108720-03	National Heart, Lung, and Blood Institute Ongoing Start: August 2013 End: July 2015	• Sickle Cell Disease • Ages 16-24	NA	• NA
A health care transition randomized trial for minority youth with special health care needs Tuchman, Lisa HRSA and MCHB HSRP20123116	Maternal and Child Health Bureau Ongoing through 2015	• Not specified	Not specified	• Not specified

Study Name Location Trial Identifier	Sponsors and Collaborators Study Status	Population Disease/Condition Age	Interventions / Groups	Primary Outcome Measures
Service transitions among youth with autism spectrum disorders Shattuck, Paul NIMH HSRP20102263	National Institutes of Health; National Institute of Mental Health Ongoing through 2014	• Autism spectrum disorder	Not specified	• Not specified
Youth with complex needs: transition to adulthood plans Rehm, Roberta S NICHD HSRP20102257	National Institute of Child Health and Human Development Completed 2012	• Complex chronic conditions	Not specified	• Not specified
Developmental Disabilities Health Care E-Toolkit McMillan, Elise Special Hope Foundation	Special Hope Foundation Ongoing	• Developmental disability	NA	• NA
Family-centered transition project Hagner, David HSRP20111046 University of New Hampshire, Institute on Disability	Maternal and Child Health Bureau Completed 2011	• Autism spectrum disorders • Age 16-18	Family-Centered transition planning model compared to usual care	• Not specified

www.ingramcontent.com/pod-product-compliance
Lightning Source LLC
Chambersburg PA
CBHW081729170526
45167CB00009B/3750

* 9 7 8 1 5 0 5 8 5 9 9 6 6 *